FOOD POSITIVITY

FOOD POSITIVITY

How to Ditch Diet Culture and Talk to Kids About Food

DIANA RICE AND DANI LEBOVITZ

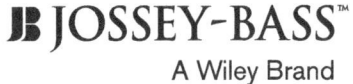

JB JOSSEY-BASS™
A Wiley Brand

Published by John Wiley & Sons, Inc., Hoboken, New Jersey.

ISBNs: 9781394335206 (Paperback), 9781394335213 (ePub), 9781394335220 (ePDF)

For general information on our other products and services or for technical support, please contact our Customer Care Department within the United States at (800) 762-2974, outside the United States at (317) 572-3993 or fax (317) 572-4002.

Wiley also publishes its books in a variety of electronic formats. Some content that appears in print may not be available in electronic formats. For more information about Wiley products, visit our web site at www.wiley.com.

Library of Congress Control Number is Available:

Cover Design and Image: Mary Navarro · Kakao Studio · www.kakaostudio.com

Printed and bound by CPI Group (UK) Ltd, Croydon, CR0 4YY

C9781394335206_120126

For every parent choosing compassion over control, curiosity over fear, and raising a generation free to trust their bodies and find joy in food.

Table of Contents

Foreword

As a pediatrician, there are so many stories and faces you never forget. These are the stories that shape your values as a doctor, mother, and advocate.

I think of the mom with her thriving 15-month-old on her lap, pleading, "Please tell me what to feed him so he gains weight. He's so scrawny." Or another parent asking me to tell his teenage daughter she's "fat" and needed to lose weight. Two very different bodies, the same fear: that their child wasn't in the "right" body.

I see this tension everywhere. Toddlers pushed to eat past fullness to "catch up." Lean kids urged to chase calories instead of balance. Children in larger bodies shamed for honoring hunger taught not to trust themselves. I've met high schoolers who binge in secret.

The result is the same: children disconnected from hunger and fullness cues, learning to see food as something to control instead of enjoy. Parents want their kids to thrive, but many feel stuck, caught in mealtime battles, weighed down by guilt, and unknowingly repeating the struggles they grew up with.

That's why this book, *Food Positivity*, is essential.

When I first connected with Diana, we talked on my podcast about how diet culture shows up in childhood. Her words resonated deeply, not just as a pediatrician but as a mom raising kids in a world that ties worth to appearance. When I came to know Dani, I saw how beautifully their strengths come together. Dani brings the joy of food exploration, the developmental insight, the playful tools parents crave. Diana brings compassion, clarity, and a deep understanding of food and body image struggles. Together, they are committed to breaking cycles and offer what parents desperately need: expertise wrapped in empathy, evidence made practical.

Parenting around food feels harder today. Most parents want to raise kids who feel positive about food and confident in their bodies, but they were never given the tools to sort through their own insecurities. Then layer on BMI charts that reduce kids to numbers and social media feeds that are packed with filtered and AI-edited bodies, "what I eat in a day" videos, misguided nutrition advice, and wellness trends disguised as health—it's no wonder families feel like they're failing.

The cost of staying stuck is steep: mealtime battles, kids disconnected from hunger cues, disordered eating that can last a lifetime, and another generation carrying the shame we hoped to leave behind.

What makes this book different is that it doesn't just focus on kids or parents; it speaks to both. *Food Positivity* helps parents reshape their own food and body stories while raising a generation free from shame. That mirrors the philosophy I share in my own work: the only way we can truly support our children is by being willing to look inward.

This book shows you how. It doesn't lecture or overwhelm. It offers real words for the moments that matter, when a child refuses dinner, begs for dessert, or says, "I'm fat." It reframes health as more than what's on a plate: nourishment, yes, but also safety, connection, and joy. With practical scripts, compassionate strategies, and evidence-based tools, it makes parenting around food and bodies less stressful while raising kids who trust themselves and grow up free from shame.

In my work, I've seen the shift when parents trust their child's body instead of controlling it. Dani and Diana's SAFE framework—Safety, Autonomy, Flexibility, and Experience—captures this. Kids don't learn to love food through pressure or shame but through safe experiences, laughter at the table, and the freedom to say "no, thank you" without fear.

As you begin to read *Food Positivity*, I hope you feel relief. Relief from micromanaging every bite. Relief from guilt. Relief in knowing that in parenting; perfection isn't the goal. Connection is. With small shifts in language and approach, you can raise kids who trust their bodies, enjoy food, and grow up free from shame.

Some of what you'll read may feel hard to hear. Especially if you grew up where food felt shameful, meals were stressful, or your body wasn't loved for what it was. Sitting with that discomfort can stir up grief, anger, or resistance. But that discomfort is not a sign you're doing it wrong. It's a sign you're breaking the cycle. The only way we change ourselves, and raise a generation free from the pain we carried, is by being willing to get uncomfortable.

My hope for every parent reading is this: may you raise kids who know food as joy, not judgment. May you raise kids who see their bodies as homes, not projects. And may you find yourself, as much as your children, set free from shame around food and bodies.

When you change the story for yourself, you change it for your children. That's the real gift of this work, and it starts here.

—Dr. Mona Amin

**Board-Certified Pediatrician, IBCLC, and
MomCreator of the Peds Doc Talk Community**

**Host of *The PedsDocTalk* Podcast, helping parents
find the confidence and calm they need**

Introduction

YOUR GRANDMOTHER HAD cigarettes and the cabbage soup diet. Your mom had Slim Fast and *Jane Fonda's Workout* at the peak of the low-fat craze. (SnackWell's, anyone?) They both had Weight Watchers, and maybe you did too.

You had Atkins, paleo, and the South Beach Diet (just reminiscing on a few. . .). And you grew up with the unshakable image of 1990s and 2000s music stars in low-rise pants with impossibly flat stomachs. And you often think of Kate Moss's infamous words ringing in the back of your mind:

"Nothing tastes as good as skinny feels."

In the last few years, it's been all about trends like "clean" eating, Whole30, keto, and intermittent fasting. And let's not forget the parade of scientifically shaky food fears—seed oils, food dyes, processed foods—on and on it goes.

The diets may change. The food rules may shift, but the message stays the same:

Your body is wrong.

Your appetite is out of control.

If you could just *fix* this pesky problem of food and your body size once and for all, your life would finally be better.

The Moment You Knew Something Was Off

You've probably felt it, the tension between what you were taught about food and bodies growing up and the way you want things to be for your kids.

Maybe it's that unsettling feeling when your child repeats a food rule you never meant to pass down, like finishing dinner before they can have dessert. Or the weight (pun not intended, but here we are) of how diet culture shows up—at the doctor's office, in schools, on their lunch trays.

Maybe you hear echoes of your own childhood at the dinner table in your home:

"Are you sure you need seconds?"

"You don't want to get fat, do you?"

Or maybe you heard:

"You're skin and bones, eat something!"

"Other kids would be grateful for this food."

And you think to yourself: *I don't want this for them. I don't want this for me either. But what on Earth do I do instead?*

You're not the only one.

Many of us are navigating the same murky water, trying to raise kids in a world where food and bodies carry way too much baggage and distract us from the things that really matter. You're ready to do things differently.

We Grew Up in Diet Culture. So Now What?

It makes sense that you're struggling. A 2022 survey by *Good Housekeeping* found that three-quarters of women have a mental list of "good" and "bad" foods.

And so, without even realizing it, we pass them down. That same survey found that 62% of parents discuss food and exercise in relation to weight with their children. We think we're helping. We all want our kids to be healthy after all! But diet culture has conditioned us to believe that certain foods are dangerous, that weight is the ultimate measure of health, and that "doing it right" means constantly policing what our children are eating.

And yet. . .the more we try to get food "right," the more we suffer.

We're all born with the ability to trust our bodies. Babies cry when they're hungry and stop when they're full. Toddlers eat three bananas one day and refuse them the next. But over time, diet culture teaches them to ignore those signals, just like it taught us.

We learn to mistrust our hunger, fear certain foods, and tie our worth to our weight. Worst of all, it takes us away from what really matters, like:

- Making memories with our kids surrounded by microwave popcorn and gummy candy on movie night
- Confidently posing for a family photo without sucking in our stomach
- Simply enjoying food without guilt

The Most Concerning Part? The Impact on Our Kids

A 2023 *Journal of the American Medical Association* meta-analysis found that 22% of children and adolescents engage in disordered eating. Another study reports that as many as 17.9% of girls and 2.4% of boys will be diagnosed with an eating disorder by young adulthood.

And we know exactly how it happens. Eating disorders are influenced by a variety of factors, but living in a culture that prioritizes some body types over others plays an enormous role. We know that we can draw a straight line from these alarming statistics back to a lifetime of being taught to ignore our *own* hunger signals.

Back to hearing that broccoli is *good* and donuts are *bad*. Back to our parents' hushed whispers of *"Don't you know how many calories are in that?"* and *"Shouldn't you eat something healthy first?"*—voices that still echo in our heads every time we reach for a snack or feed our kids.

The Parenting Paradox: Freedom vs. Fear

We want to raise kids who feel free to be exactly who they are, to dress how they want, to love who they love, and to chase their dreams.

But when it comes to food and their bodies? That freedom feels terrifying. Because we've been taught that letting go of food rules means letting go of their future.

That if we don't control what they eat. . .

. . .they'll eat nothing but junk.

. . .they'll be bullied for their size.

. . .they'll be unhealthy, or worse.

We want them to be well-nourished, of course. But we also live in a world that tells us fatness is a fast track to disease and early death (which isn't true by the way—more on this in Chapter 1).

So how do we let go of control without feeling like we're setting them up for struggle? How do we raise kids to trust their bodies when we've spent a lifetime being told we can't trust ours? How can we shift from control to support when we don't even know what that support is supposed to look like?

The Tipping Point

Thankfully, things are changing. More and more people, including medical organizations, researchers, and everyday parents, are questioning the dangers of diet culture. Athletes, musicians, actors, and influencers who don't fit the traditional beauty mold are taking up space, sharing their stories, and offering our kids the role models we never had.

And, we have research on our side. Studies are clear that the way we talk about these subjects in our kids' early years affects their long-term relationships with food and their bodies. We also know that body shape and size are mostly determined by genetics and environmental factors, not the "hard work and dedication" touted by diet culture. And we've learned that the number-one predictor of weight gain in both children and adults is, ironically, trying to lose weight in the first place.

But most importantly, we're finally realizing our power as parents. We're the first generation with the opportunity to break these cycles—to say *enough* to the food guilt, the body shame, the relentless pursuit of thinness disguised as "health."

What if we redefined what food means, not just for our kids, but for ourselves too?

Diet culture has stolen so much joy from eating, reducing it to numbers, rules, and guilt. It's time to take that joy back, for our kids, and for ourselves. It's time for **Food Positivity**.

What Is Food Positivity?

Every parent wants their kids to grow up healthy, eat a variety of foods, and feel good in their bodies. But so many of us find ourselves stuck—in dinner battles, negotiations over sugar, or the quiet fear that our children will inherit the same struggles with food and body image that we grew up with.

Food Positivity is more than how we feed kids—*it's how we raise them*. It's the decision to make mealtimes a place of trust instead of conflict, joy instead of guilt, and connection instead of control. Instead of focusing on rules, pressure, or perfection, Food Positivity supports the whole child—body, mind, and spirit. It gives parents practical tools to make mealtimes calmer *today* while raising kids who explore food with curiosity, trust their bodies, and eat well for *life*.

Our mission is simple: to help families break cycles of shame and guilt so the next generation can inherit something better—*a relationship with food and their bodies rooted in safety, trust, joy, and whole-child well-being.*

A Fresh Perspective: More Than Just "Food Neutrality"

You may have heard of Food Neutrality, which teaches that all foods have equal moral value, meaning you're neither "good" or "bad" based on what you eat. It removes those labels altogether.

Food Positivity takes it further. It's not just about what we take *away*, it's about what we *add*:

Instead of only removing guilt, we create joy.

Instead of avoiding pressure, we build confidence.

Instead of only treating food as fuel, we embrace it as connection, culture, and learning.

Food Positivity isn't just about eating, it's about raising kids who:

- Trust their bodies
- Feel safe exploring new foods
- Enjoy food without guilt
- Develop a healthy relationship with eating for life

Food Positivity is both an approach parents can take and a life skill children grow into—one that makes food a source of safety, trust, connection, and joy. It nurtures whole-child well-being so kids grow up nourished, confident, curious, and resilient against food and body shame.

The Science Behind Food Positivity

If you've ever tried to get a toddler to put their shoes on, you probably know kids don't learn positive habits through control, fear, or shame.

Food Positivity isn't just some "feel-good" parenting philosophy. It's grounded in decades of research on child development, psychology, neuroscience, education, and nutrition. But you don't need to be an expert to use it. What you'll find in this book are simple, practical ways to put it into action—from the words you say at the table to how you respond when your child comments on someone's body to the way you model your own relationship with food. It's evidence-based, and it works.

But honestly? It also just makes sense. Kids learn best when they watch us model healthy behaviors. When they get to explore and learn through play. And when they feel like they have a say in their own choices. Food should be fun, not forced. And most importantly, kids thrive when they trust themselves, not when every meal turns into a battle over bites.

Does This Mean Nutrition Doesn't Matter?

Nope. Actually, it's the opposite. But as you'll see, *what* you feed matters, but *how* you feed makes all the difference.

Food Positivity is about recognizing that nutrition *does* matter, so much so that we want to teach kids about food and nutrition in a way that supports them for a lifetime. What we're after is kids who become adults with the ability to think, "Eh, I don't really think a donut would feel very good right now" or "Hey, I could really go for a salad!" without the food police whispering in their ears either way.

Research shows us how early food experiences shape lifelong well-being. The way we teach kids about food today, whether they feel pressure, joy, or guilt, affects:

- The variety of foods they eat
- How open they are to trying new foods
- Whether they learn to listen to their bodies (or override their hunger cues)
- Their sense of connection and belonging at the table

Food Positivity supports whole-child well-being by recognizing that if we want to raise healthy kids from the inside out, we can't just focus on *what* they eat; we have to transform *how* they experience food.

Meet Your Guides

We are so excited and honored to be part of your parenting journey. Between the two of us, we've spent more than 35 years helping parents raise kids with a healthy, happy relationship with food. Dani is a dietitian who specializes in early childhood development. Her passion is creating food education for kids, and she has spent years teaching families how to approach food with curiosity and confidence. Diana is a dietitian and Certified Intuitive Eating Counselor who specializes in helping parents untangle their own food and body beliefs so they can raise kids without the same struggles.

But beyond our professional credentials, we're both moms who know firsthand how hard it is to navigate food and body talk in a world that's constantly telling us we're doing it wrong. We've seen the harms of diet culture in our own lives and the lives of the families we work with. We know that parents aren't *trying* to pass down food and body guilt; they just don't know what to do instead. That's why we wrote this book: to help you step out of the cycle of food shame, weight fears, and impossible food rules and into something better.

How to Use This Book

Each chapter opens with a story from parents who've inspired this resource. We hope you'll see yourself in their experiences and realize you're not the only one trying to figure all this out.

Here's what you'll find:

Part I: Where our food and body beliefs come from and how awareness helps us change.

Part II: How kids think, grow, and form food and body beliefs, so you can meet them where they are.

Part III: How to unpack what you've inherited and create a shame-free food environment that reflects your family's values.

Part IV: Real-life tools and scripts to handle those tricky food and body moments with more calm and confidence.

Part V: How to take Food Positivity beyond your home—to schools, healthcare, and the next generation growing up free from shame.

Throughout the book, you'll also hear from experts who are putting this approach into practice every day with their clients, patients, and families.

And since we're pretty big on *experiential learning*, every chapter ends with **One Simple Step** you can put into practice today.

You'll also get access to our companion website with bonus handouts, full chapter references, and a downloadable workbook called **Your Food Positivity Practice: A Guided Playbook for Real-Life Parenting**. At the end of each chapter, we'll point you to the matching workbook page to keep the learning going.

Access All Companion Materials Here
Scan the QR code to find:

- Your Food Positivity Practice: A Guided Playbook for Real-Life Parenting
- Bonus handouts and tools
- Full chapter references and glossary

(Once you've scanned it, bookmark the page so you can find it easily as you read.)

Breaking the Cycle Starts Here

We know it's not easy. Undoing years (and maybe even decades) of food guilt, body shame, and rigid food rules isn't something that happens overnight.

You're not just feeding your kids.
You're rebuilding trust in food, in bodies, and in yourself.
You're breaking cycles that have shaped generations.

You're giving your child something you never had: the freedom to grow up feeling safe, confident, and at home in their own body. And that's powerful.

This journey won't be perfect. And that's okay. Because raising intuitive eaters who trust their own bodies isn't about getting every meal "right." It's about showing up, learning, and unlearning—one step at a time.

You don't have to do this alone.

We're here to help you rethink old narratives, navigate tricky moments, and give you the tools you need to raise a child who feels at peace with food and their body—for *life*.

You're here because something in you *knows* there's a better way.

This book will help you find it. Let's get started.

One Simple Step

Think back to something an adult said to you about food when you were younger. Do you still hear that voice in your head today? Did it help you eat "better," or does it bring up guilt, shame, or confusion?

Now ask yourself: What voices do you want your child to hear in their head when they grow up?

Let that question guide you as you read this book.

Your Food Positivity Practice

Exploring My Food & Body Story: *Where My Beliefs Begin*

PART

I

What We've Inherited and the Foundations for Change

1

Understanding Health and the Impact of Diet Culture

Sometimes I look at my daughter next to her thinner friends with a knot in my stomach. I tell myself she's healthy and strong but definitely worry she's "too big." I grew up with comments about my portion sizes, warnings not to "let myself go," and relatives who were always on one diet or another. I don't want my daughter to feel that kind of shame, but I can already feel how it shapes the way I see her.

—Tara

HAS THERE EVER been a moment in your parenting journey when you thought, *There has got to be a better way?*

Maybe it was when your child told you their snack wasn't "healthy," and you wondered where they picked that up.

Or when the pediatrician mentioned your child's weight and you were instantly transported back to being eight years old, hearing the same comments about yourself.

Or maybe it was that moment at the dinner table when you heard yourself say, "No dessert until you finish your veggies," and thought, *I sound just like my mom.*

3

Whatever sparked it, you felt it—the pull to do things differently and break the cycle. To do that, we first need to take a critical look at the messages about health, food, and bodies that got us here.

What If We've Had the Wrong Definition of Health All Along?

Most of us learned about "health" long before we understood the word. It came bundled with food rules, weight talk, and labels about "good" and "bad" choices.

- Being healthy meant being thin.
- It meant eating "right" and avoiding "junk."
- It meant not gaining too much weight.

And without even realizing it, we've carried those ideas into snack time, onto our dinner plates, and into the way we talk to our kids.

Those ideas didn't come from out of nowhere. They came from **diet culture**, a system of beliefs that links body ideals with health and worth, promotes weight loss both necessary for health and a moral obligation, and teaches us that only certain ways of eating are "right." It fuels shame, disordered eating, and disconnection from our bodies' natural cues by keeping us focused on our body sizes instead of living life to its fullest.

And it's not just personal. It's a system that harms people in larger bodies, women, people of color, LGBTQ+ folks, and those with disabilities most of all.

But the real question is, are those messages actually helping us raise healthier kids? Think back to how they made you feel growing up. Did they leave you feeling confident or ashamed? Did they build trust in your body or teach you to second-guess it?

Chances are, they didn't lead to lifelong joy around food. They led to guilt, fear, and a complicated relationship with eating. And these messages don't just shape the way *we* think about food—they influence our kids. Studies show that children exposed to parental dieting, weight-focused conversations, or food rules are more likely to develop disordered eating, body dissatisfaction, and lower self-esteem.

And the scariest part? Kids internalize these messages *young*.

- By age 3, children begin to associate larger bodies with negative traits.
- By age 5, they start worrying about their own body size.
- By age 9, many kids have already experimented with dieting.

This is why the way we talk about food and bodies matters, every single day. So, what if we stopped repeating those messages and started rewriting them?

Health ≠ Weight

Most of us grew up equating health with a number, the one on the scale, the one on the growth chart, or the one on the Body Mass Index (BMI) report that came home from school. But here's the truth: **Health is *not* a body size**.

Instead of teaching kids to monitor their weight or earn their food, we can help them build skills they'll use for life: listening to hunger and fullness cues, trying new foods with curiosity, and learning to respect their body as it grows. We can create environments where food is joyful, mealtimes are safe and predictable, and we move our bodies because of how good it feels, not how many calories it burns. We can model self-care and body respect for ourselves, showing our kids that health isn't a number but a lifelong practice of caring for our bodies with joy, compassion, and trust.

EXPERT INSIGHT: Health Is More Than a Number: A Weight Inclusive Researcher Perspective

Dawn Clifford, PhD, RD Professor of Health Sciences, Northern Arizona University

Over the last few decades, health and fitness professionals have tried to "fix" chronic disease with "just lose weight" messaging, which completely negates the very complex health puzzle.

(*continued*)

(*continued*)

In a lot of ways, telling someone to lose weight actually increases stress and worsens health. Now we know that weight is a terrible indicator of health and that health is impacted by many factors outside of the individual's control such as trauma, poverty, food insecurity, unsafe neighborhoods, stigma, and discrimination.

Weight is one of the many factors that make us diverse humans—just like height, hair color, skin, and eye color. Our genetics largely drive body weight, shape, and size. Instead of shaming people for their bodies, we need to celebrate size diversity.

Instead of focusing on changing your child's weight, focus on loving them just the way they are. Teach them that every *BODY* is unique and worthy of love and acceptance.

The Problem with BMI

What do you think of when you hear the phrases "healthy weight," "overweight," and "obese"?

In medical terms, these phrases refer to categories outlined by the BMI, a chart that labels weight status as "healthy," "overweight," or "obese." But the BMI was never designed to measure individual health. It was created in the 1830s by Belgian statistician Adolphe Quetelet to study averages of "the normal man"—white, European men, to be exact. It doesn't account for gender, age, ethnicity, muscle mass, mental health, or lifestyle. Yet, for decades, it's been used as a gatekeeper for healthcare, insurance, and even school report cards.

Thankfully, things are shifting, and even the American Medical Association acknowledged the BMI's limitations in 2023. But many of us still hold the belief that smaller bodies = healthier bodies.

Research tells a different story: People in larger bodies can be metabolically healthy, and people in smaller bodies can have the same health concerns we blame on weight like diabetes and heart disease. A major meta-analysis (a study of many other studies) by the Centers for Disease Control (CDC) in 2013 found something surprising: The lowest risk of death was in the "overweight" group, and the highest risk was the "underweight" group. And the "healthy weight" group? Their risk was practically identical to those in the "obese" group.

So why does this matter for parents? Because when we use BMI or weight as our main health marker, we're not looking at the whole child and we risk missing what's really important, a child's emotional well-being, growth pattern, and relationship with food.

Words About Weight Matter

Terms like "overweight" and "obese" are common in healthcare but carry stigma and reinforce weight bias.

"Obese" comes from a Latin word meaning "to have eaten until fat," which is misleading and inaccurate—bodies come in many shapes and sizes for reasons that have little to do with what we eat. While words like "overweight," "obese," and "healthy weight" are common in medicine, research, and everyday conversations, this suggests there's one "right" weight for health. But research shows health can't be measured by a single number.

Throughout this book, we'll use more respectful, inclusive, and accurate language that affirms all bodies such as "small," "large," "thin," and "fat" because bodies don't need fixing, but the words we use to talk about them do.

What *Real* Health Looks Like

When we strip away diet culture's influence, health looks very different than what most of us were taught.

The World Health Organization (WHO) defines health as, "A state of complete physical, mental, and social well-being, not merely the absence of disease or infirmity."

That's the vision we want for our kids, a whole-child approach to health that asks:

- **Physical well-being:** Are they growing, sleeping, and playing well?
- **Mental and emotional health:** Do they feel happy, supported, and resilient?

- **Social well-being:** Do they feel safe and connected?
- **Body trust:** Can they recognize and respond to their hunger, fullness, and emotions?

When we look at the whole child, it's clear that raising "healthy" kids isn't just about controlling what goes on their plates. It's about fostering an environment that supports *your* child's individual needs and helps them develop the skills they'll need to thrive.

Zoom Out: The Bigger Forces at Play

Once we let go of the idea that health is just about weight, we can start to see the bigger picture. That our kids' well-being is shaped by far more than what's on their plate or how much they move their bodies.

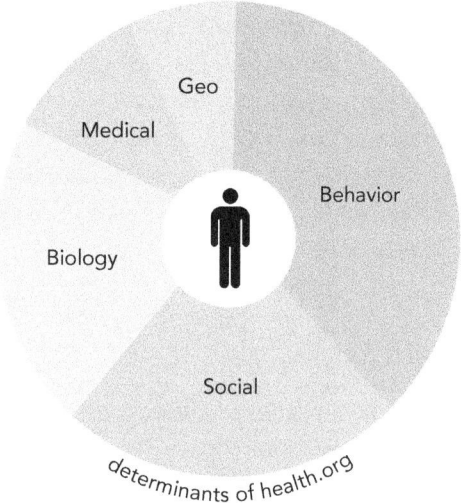

Research shows that only about 30–40% of health outcomes are shaped by individual behaviors (like what we eat, how we move, if we smoke, and whether we wear our seatbelt). The other 60–70% are influenced by factors outside of our direct control and come from the world around us. These are the opportunities, stressors, and access to resources that make up daily life known as the Social Determinants of Health (SDoH).

> When we understand these bigger forces, we can release some of the pressure we put on ourselves and our kids to "get it right" with every bite.

Social Determinants of Health: If Health Were a House

Instead of thinking of health as a personal responsibility, think of your family's health like a house. A safe, sturdy house keeps your family protected, but its strength doesn't depend on willpower; it depends on when you build it, where you build it, and the materials and conditions available to build and maintain it. Below are the "building materials" in real life:

Blueprint = genetics + biology

> Every house starts with a blueprint. Our inherited traits and body functions shape the frame we're working with. Some frames are naturally sturdy; others need extra care and maintenance.

Daily upkeep = individual behavior

> What you eat, how you move, your sleep, and other habits are like routine house maintenance. They matter, but they can't fix a crumbling foundation or a leaky roof on their own.

Foundation = social circumstances

> Education, job opportunities, income, race, and ethnicity, culture, social circles, and access to safe, affordable food form the base your house sits on. A strong foundation keeps everything steady. Cracks, like poverty, discrimination, or food insecurity, make it harder for kids to thrive.

Windows + doors = healthcare access

> Compassionate, affordable, quality healthcare—together with health literacy—are like having working windows and doors. They let you get help when you need it. If care is too far away, too expensive, or not culturally sensitive, it's like being locked out in a storm.

Roof + yard = environment

Safe neighborhoods, clean air, nearby grocery stores, and parks make up the roof and yard that protect and support your family. A strong roof keeps out harm and a safe yard gives kids space to play and grow. A leak in the roof or hazards in the yard—such as crime, pollution, or lack of grocery stores— invite stress and hardship, making it harder for kids to feel secure and thrive.

When we focus only on "personal responsibility," we miss these massive drivers of health. It's like blaming parents for a leaky roof without acknowledging that they were given faulty materials, no budget for repairs, and a storm overhead.

Health Is Not Just About Choices, It's About Access

Most of us were taught that health is as simple as "eat well and exercise." But real life isn't that simple.

Because if health were *only* about making "better choices," then what about the 47 million people in the United States who don't always know where their next meal is coming from? What about families living in neighborhoods where fresh groceries are too expensive or just not available?

Here's what we need to name out loud:

- **Food insecurity:** You can't "choose healthy" if there's no food to choose from.
- **Food deserts:** Some communities don't have affordable grocery stores, or any grocery store at all, just fast food or corner stores.
- **Poverty and racism:** Families in lower-income or marginalized communities face higher rates of illness, not because they're making worse choices but because they have fewer resources, less access to safe places to play, and fewer trusted doctors.
- **Racism is a health risk:** Yep, you read that right. Experiencing discrimination raises stress hormones, which can lead to high blood pressure, heart disease, and mental health struggles.

- **Weight stigma hurts health:** When people are judged for their body size, they're less likely to seek care and more likely to face chronic stress, disordered eating, and poorer health outcomes.

When we put the full weight of health on "personal responsibility," we end up blaming parents and kids for things they can't control instead of fixing the systems that make health harder for some families than others.

The Role of Trauma and Food Insecurity

Trauma is a powerful force that can shape how kids relate to food. Adverse Childhood Experiences (ACEs) are a clinical measure of potentially traumatic events—such as abuse, neglect, or household food insecurity, exposure to addiction, or a caregiver's mental illness—and leave a lasting imprint on a child's brain and body.

"Child abuse and neglect is the single most preventable cause of mental illness, the single most common cause of drug and alcohol abuse, and a significant contributor to leading causes of death such as diabetes, heart disease, cancer, stroke, and suicide."
—Bessel A. van der Kolk, *The Body Keeps the Score*

Research shows that higher ACE scores increase the risk for chronic diseases later in life, including diabetes, heart disease, depression, and, yes, disordered eating. Kids who experience ACEs are also more likely to struggle with emotional regulation and may turn to food as a way to cope.

And here's the kicker: Food insecurity itself is considered an ACE. Studies show that food insecurity is linked to behaviors like:

- Hoarding or sneaking food
- Eating past fullness because they don't know when their next meal will come
- Distrust of their hunger and fullness cues

■ Feeling deep shame around food, even when there's plenty available

When kids grow up in environments where their basic needs aren't consistently met, these survival patterns stay with them. Even when life becomes more stable, these patterns continue to shape how they approach food and their bodies for years to come.

And if *you* grew up in these circumstances, it's common to feel torn: stuck between old food-scarcity beliefs and the desire to give your kids a calmer, more peaceful relationship with eating.

Two Common (but Opposite) Patterns We've Seen

We often think about how diet culture shows up in homes where parents have strict opinions about "healthy" eating and avoiding weight gain.

But there's another pattern we don't talk about enough. Some parents, overwhelmed by financial stress, mental health struggles, or just trying to get by, don't have the bandwidth to support kids with positive food leadership. It's not that they don't care; it's just that fast food and packaged snacks are a lifeline when a family is just trying to get by.

In both highly controlled and unstructured homes (what we'll explore in Chapter 12 as authoritarian versus permissive/neglectful parenting), kids don't grow up with the supportive structures they need. Some may feel guilty about their food choices or bounce between restriction and binging while others blame the convenience foods of their childhood for their food struggles as adults. But in both cases, the real issue is missing out on the support they needed to nourish themselves well from the start.

We're not blaming parents here—in both cases, parents do their best with the tools and resources they have. Many are carrying their own food and body struggles, often passed down from the generations before them. And some families don't fall into either extreme, but diet culture still crept in later through friends, media, or healthcare.

However it showed up, most of us are navigating some version of a world where we didn't have the support we needed.

Parent Reflection

Pause for a moment and notice how you feel after reading this chapter. Diet culture, systemic barriers, trauma, and food access can feel heavy—and that's okay.

You might feel sadness, anger, or even guilt as you think about your own childhood or your parenting journey so far. Every one of these feelings is valid. And you don't have to have it all figured out today to start changing the story.

Bringing It Home

So if you've ever thought, *There has got to be a better way*, you're absolutely right. The messages many of us grew up with about food, bodies, and health weren't neutral—and they often weren't grounded in science either. They were shaped by diet culture and systems that left us anxious and confused, not healthier.

This isn't about blaming the past; it's about noticing where those unhelpful patterns came from so you can choose how to rewrite these messages for *your* family.

And the good news is, you've already started. Just pausing to notice is a huge step. Every time you offer food without pressure, respect your child's hunger and fullness cues, or speak about bodies with curiosity instead of criticism, you're supporting your kids' whole well-being and helping them develop the skills they need to thrive.

While you can't erase weight stigma, fix food deserts, or stop every harmful comment your child hears on the playground—you *can* create a home that feels safe, predictable, and shame-free. Over time, these small choices become a protective shield your child carries with them, helping them sort through all the mixed messages about health, food, and their bodies.

One Simple Step

Notice when the word "healthy" comes up this week in your thoughts, in conversation, or in something your child hears.

Pause and ask yourself:

"What do I really mean by healthy here?"

You don't need to change anything yet. Just start noticing. That awareness alone is a powerful step toward rewriting what health means in *your* family.

Your Food Positivity Practice

Redefining Health: *Making Sense of What I Learned Growing Up*

2

Unpacking the Roots of Diet Culture in Our Food System

In fourth grade, my class had a health unit about "better choices." The teacher explained that brown rice was healthier than white because it had more fiber and that it was an "easy swap." So that night, I told my mom we should switch to brown rice. She scoffed and said she's been eating white rice her whole life and certainly wasn't going to change that now. I knew there was no use arguing with her, so every time we had white rice after that I just ate as little as I could, even though I often wanted more. It was easier than feeling like I was eating something unhealthy.

—Lina

THINK BACK TO your childhood. By now, you've likely started noticing the food and body messages you grew up with, the comments, the rules, and the quiet lessons that still live rent free in your brain. Your mom sighing that she "shouldn't" eat dessert, a health lesson that introduced you to counting calories. At the time, these messages felt normal. They were just. . .how people talked about food.

But now we can see how those messages shaped us. How they made us feel like we had to shrink, control, and second-guess our hunger. And the last thing we want is to pass on that same burden to our kids.

Diet culture didn't start with us.

It's been passed down for generations, like an old family recipe no one asked for but everyone kept on making. Let's step back in time and explore the history of diet culture and how it shaped the food system we are raising our kids in today.

Parent Reflection

Before we jump into the next few chapters, we want to give you a heads-up. Some of what you're about to read might feel uncomfortable, and you may find yourself thinking: "Wait, what does this have to do with how I talk to my kids about food?"

Over the next several pages we'll trace the roots of food and body shame and how it became so normalized. We'll touch on privilege, bias, and the ways our food system has shaped what's considered "healthy" or "good."

This information can feel heavy, especially if you realize you've benefited from some of these systems or if you've been harmed by them. But this chapter isn't about blame; it's about connecting the dots so we can stop passing along lessons that don't serve us or our kids.

Where Did These Food and Body Rules Come From?

For most of history, food was about survival, tradition, and connection. People ate what was available and their foodways (what they ate, the way they prepared food, and the cultural role those foods played in daily life) were passed down and carried their culture forward.

But when European settlers colonized lands around the world, they brought more than their food; they brought ideas about what foods and bodies they believed to be "civilized" or acceptable.

It's important to note that by "European settlers," we're talking mostly about Northern and Western Europeans from Great Britain; White Anglo-Saxon Protestants who were both Caucasian and Christian.

This is an important distinction because, as you'll see, not all Europeans were considered part of this "civilized" group. Southern and Eastern Europeans, such as Italians, Jews, Ukrainians, Greeks, and others, were excluded for decades, which shaped how whiteness and privilege were defined in the United States.

As medicine, public health, and nutrition science began to take shape in the United States, these biases formed their foundation. And because Western medicine dismissed, exploited, and excluded people of color, many of these inaccurate beliefs became "baked in" to the way we define nutritious food and healthy bodies even today.

From stigmatizing bodies and marginalizing traditional diets to medical recommendations built on racist assumptions, these deeply rooted systemic biases continue to reinforce inequities, widen health disparities, and perpetuate inaccurate "health" information and nutrition recommendations. Together we'll look at the history of how the biases that shape modern diet culture evolved in a way that's never really been about health.

How Bias Shaped "Healthy Eating"

Once you see these patterns, you can't unsee them. Here's how history still shows up in our idea of "healthy" foods today:

- **"Balanced plates" that all look the same:** MyPlate-style visuals often leave out traditional dishes like curries, tamales, stir-fried noodles, and stews that don't fit neatly into sections.
- **Western food guides as the gold standard:** Many nutrition recommendations were created for white, middle-class families with access to certain foods, leaving out what was available or affordable for other communities.
- **Dismissing cultural staples:** Calling white rice, plantains, or flatbreads "unhealthy" ignores how they've nourished families

(*continued*)

(*continued*)

for generations including cultures with longer life expectancies than the United States.

- **Marginalized to mainstream:** Watermelon was once weaponized as a racist stereotype to shame Black Americans, even though it was a nourishing crop that symbolized freedom and economic independence. And bagels and pizza, once dismissed as "foreign" foods tied to poverty, were kept alive by immigrant communities until the rest of America caught on. Today, all three are loved but rarely do we pause to honor the history and resilience behind them.
- **The "Superfood" label cycle:** Traditional foods like quinoa, chia, and turmeric were once devalued or associated with lower social status and dismissed as "peasant foods" and then rebranded in Western wellness culture as expensive "superfoods," often pricing out the communities who grew and ate them first.

Recognizing these patterns helps us appreciate the rich culture behind our food and teach our kids that there are many ways to eat well.

1600s: Colonization and Early Food Systems

When Northern and Western European settlers arrived in North America, they brought food traditions centered on breads and porridges, salted and smoked meats, butter and cheese, and preserving fruits and vegetables through pickling and fermentation.

Indigenous communities already had sophisticated seasonal food systems that shaped their cultures and what grew in the region. Their diets were rich in corn, beans, squash, foraged plants, and wild game. But colonists often dismissed these ways of eating as "primitive." This judgment was the start of a food hierarchy, where European ways of eating were seen as "better" and Indigenous foods were devalued. This wasn't just about food; it was about power and control.

1700s: The Transatlantic Slave Trade and Food Oppression

The transatlantic slave trade added another layer to this hierarchy, built on forced labor, deprivation, and resilience. Enslaved Africans were stripped of their traditional foodways and given small amounts of unfamiliar foods such as cornmeal, salted meat or fish, and sometimes molasses—just enough to keep them alive.

But many enslaved people carried seeds across the ocean, hiding them in their hair or clothing, and planted gardens on the edges of plantations, often called "slave gardens." They grew okra, yams, cowpeas, watermelon, and greens. These foods not only nourished their bodies and preserved their culture but also slowly shaped the food systems of the very plantations where they were forced to work, becoming staples of Southern cuisine.

Late 1800s to Early 1900s: Assimilation and "Americanization"

Fast-forward to the late 1800s when waves of Eastern and Southern European immigrants arrived in the United States. Each community brought their own cultural foodways including pasta, pierogi, borscht, baklava, gefilte fish, and sausages to name a few. But stigmatization, marginalization, and active policy-driven assimilation encouraged "Americanized" meals to reshape immigrant eating habits.

1900s: The Rise of "Healthy Eating" as a Moral Standard

By the early 1900s, nutrition science was becoming formalized, with the U.S. Department of Agriculture (USDA) offering some of the first national dietary guidelines. But this wasn't just about nutrients; it was about morality.

Eugenics, the now discredited belief that society could improve by eliminating "undesirable" traits, shaped early public health campaigns. "Eating right" and personal health were framed as civic virtues and signs of being a "good American." Physical strength, productivity, and patriotism—especially during World War I—were tied to what and how people ate.

Immigrants were pressured to abandon their cultural foodways, labeling their traditional dishes as "too spicy," "greasy," or simply

"unhealthy" and "uncivilized." Nutrition became a tool for assimilation and was deeply intertwined with racial hierarchies and the belief
in body superiority. "Healthy eating" became less about nourishment
and more about proving you were disciplined, moral, and worthy. This
idea evolved into today's "healthism," today, where health is seen as
both a personal responsibility and a measure of someone's value.

**Farmers' bulletin United States. Dept. of Agriculture 1917: What the
Body Needs**

4   FARMERS' BULLETIN 808.

THE DAY'S FOOD.

A man who does fairly hard muscular* work would be likely to
get the food which his body needs if supplied daily with such a
combination of foods as the following:

1¼ pounds of bread, having about the same food value as 1 pound of such cereal
    preparations as wheat or rye flour, oatmeal, cornmeal, rice, etc.
2 ounces, or ¼ cup, of butter, oil, meat drippings, or other fat.
2 ounces, or ¼ cup, of sugar; or ⅓ cup of honey, or sirup, or an equivalent
    amount of other sweet.

1950s to 1970s: Diet Culture Goes Mainstream

By the 1950s, diet culture wasn't just a fad; it became part of how
people defined "good health" and moral worth. Public health messaging said that health was an individual responsibility and that thinness
was its ultimate proof. Government campaigns focused on "fixing"
health through personal choice, ignoring systemic barriers like poverty, racism, and lack of access to fresh food.

Around that same time, advertisements equated thinness with success, beauty, and self-control. These ideas didn't just shame people
about their bodies; they also reinforced racist and classist beliefs about
which bodies—and which communities—were "acceptable" or "right"
(think thin, white, and middle-class).

By the early 1960s, American housewife Jean Nidetch began
organizing support meetings in her living room with friends who were
trying to lose weight together. By 1968, her company Weight Watchers
went public, and dieting became a full-on, mainstream movement,
selling weight loss as a way to gain social approval.

The low-fat craze, or "War on Fat," came right behind it. Suddenly,
foods like nuts, avocados, and whole-fat dairy, once staples, were now
labeled and grouped into the "unhealthy" category.

Thinness became *the* goal. Food was something to control. And if you didn't? Well, Nidetch once famously said, "It's choice—not chance—that determines your destiny." Translation? If you don't control your own weight, that's a *you* problem.

1960s President's Physical Fitness ad linking modern conveniences and food pleasure to moral decline

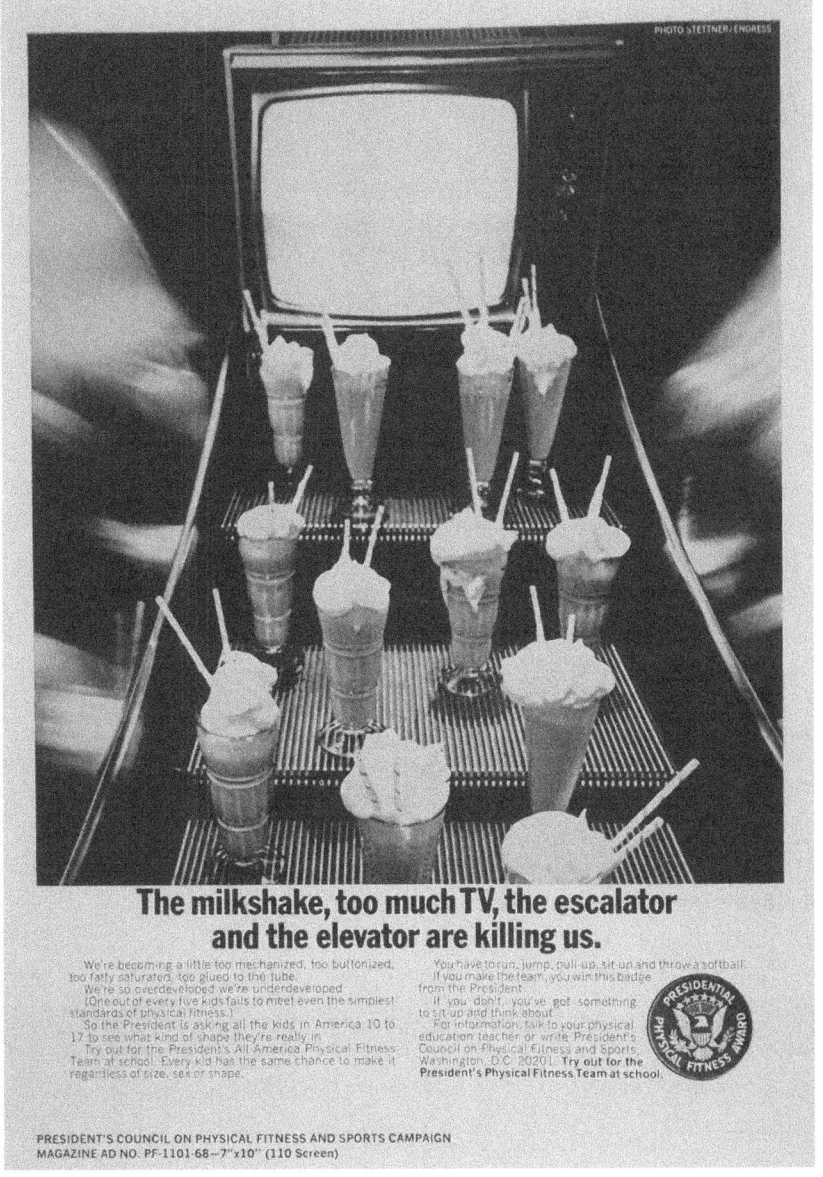

PRESIDENT'S COUNCIL ON PHYSICAL FITNESS AND SPORTS CAMPAIGN
MAGAZINE AD NO. PF-1101-68—7"x10" (110 Screen)

1980s to 2000s: Dieting Becomes Big Business

By the 1980s, dieting had turned into a multibillion-dollar industry. Everywhere you looked, there were calorie counters, SlimFast shakes, portion rules, and "good versus bad food" lists. From magazine covers promising "flat abs in 10 days" to Jane Fonda advising us to snack on sweet potatoes when a candy craving hit, food rules were the new norm.

Then in 1998, the BMI categories used to classify people's health by weight were quietly adjusted, literally overnight. Millions of Americans woke up in a new "overweight" or "obese" category. But this wasn't a sudden health crisis; it was a shift of the goalposts that opened the door for the diet industry to sell even more weight-loss programs and products to "fix" this so-called problem.

And just when the low-fat craze started to lose steam, the low-carb and "clean-eating" trends took over—same guilt, different branding.

2010s to Today: Diet Culture Gets a Makeover

Enter the influencer era. Social media gave diet culture a shiny new filter and called it "wellness." Instead of magazine covers and TV commercials, we now get "what I eat in a day" videos, detox tea ads, and color-coded bento box lunches.

It's still the same message: control your body, control your food, prove your worth. Only now it's coming from influencers you follow and trust instead of credentialed experts.

The Lasting Legacy of Food Stigma

Generations of families were pressured to abandon their cultural foods in the name of "health." Women, especially, carried the burden of shrinking their bodies by counting calories, exercising to "earn" food, and staying busy with self-control over joy.

Today, parents still feel judged for feeding their kids meals that don't look like the Western "healthy plate" model, despite that those foods have nourished their families for generations. And we're still told to "just eat healthy," even while living in a food system that makes fresh, nourishing food easy to access for some families and far harder for others.

Access Matters More Than "Making Better Choices"

If you've ever felt like feeding your family is harder than it should be, you're not imagining it. The idea that people just need to "make better choices" ignores a glaring truth: not everyone *has* the same choices. How can you choose fresh vegetables if your closest store sells only chips and soda? Or when strawberries cost twice as much as cookies?

This isn't about willpower; it's about access. For decades, entire communities, especially Black and Brown neighborhoods, were boxed out of affordable, fresh food options by unfair policies like redlining.

Redlining was a racist practice that literally drew red lines around certain neighborhoods on maps and denied them loans and investments. As a result, grocery stores avoided those areas, while fast-food chains and liquor stores moved in. Government food programs tried to help but often fell short of providing the nourishing foods families needed to thrive.

Even today, many parents are doing their best while juggling food deserts, sky-high prices, and very little time to cook due to the stresses of work and life. And still, parents are told, "just feed your kids better."

What's often missing from this conversation is that research about the "harms" of processed food rarely accounts for the bigger picture— poverty, time scarcity, stress, and systemic barriers—as well as why certain communities rely on these foods more often in the first place.

People rely on processed food because it's what's available, affordable, and realistic in their lives. This isn't about poor choices. It's about a system that was never built with every family in mind.

And while we are highlighting the way these access issues historically disproportionately affected communities of color, families across all racial and cultural backgrounds who face poverty or live in under-resourced areas experience the same barriers.

So if you've ever grabbed frozen pizza, hit the drive-thru after work, or felt guilty that your child's lunch isn't Instagram-worthy, you're not failing. The system just wasn't designed to make this easy.

Bringing It Home

By now you've seen that diet culture isn't new; it's been shaping food, bodies, and parenting for centuries. And while learning this history may be unsettling, it helps explain why so many of us feel guilty about food, stressed about feeding our kids, and pressured to "get it right." And awareness is power.

Looking at the roots of diet culture helps us see it for what it is and gives us a chance to stop repeating old patterns. We can teach our kids that food isn't something to fear or control but something to connect with and enjoy.

And the best part is, there is no one-size-fits-all! When food is about connection instead of control, you can celebrate your cultural foodways and raise your kids with what you want them to learn about food.

One Simple Step

Choose one cultural or family food that diet culture has labeled as "unhealthy" or "bad."

Serve it with pride and notice what it brings beyond nutrition: joy, comfort, connection, heritage.

Then ask yourself: "What would it look like to teach my child that this food belongs on their plate, exactly as it is? How would that feel for you (and for them)?"

Your Food Positivity Practice

Noticing Our Food Beliefs: *Bringing Hidden Messages Into the Light*

3

The Pursuit of Thinness: How Diet Culture Shapes Our Relationship with Our Bodies

Classmates and relatives always commented on my size, but no one seemed to notice how often I skipped meals or secretly threw food away. I managed to lose weight a few times, but I was never small enough to escape the comments. Even now, I get anxious eating in front of other people, even when they've been nothing but kind to me.

—Alex

MAYBE YOU'VE CAUGHT yourself wishing your body looked different, even while trying to teach your kids to love theirs. Or maybe you've felt a pang of fear seeing your child's body change, wondering if you should be doing something about it, even though you don't want to repeat the shame you grew up with.

If that's where you are right now, you're in good company. So many parents feel this tension, wanting to do better for your kids while still wrestling with the beliefs you've absorbed about bodies.

This chapter explores how those body ideals were formed, how they became tied to morality and worth, and how they still shape the messages our kids hear today. We'll look at the harm these messages cause and start practicing a new way of thinking so your kids grow up feeling safe and at home in their bodies.

Bridging Food and Body Oppression

In many premodern societies, larger bodies—especially women's bodies—were celebrated. In times when food was scarce, a fuller figure often signaled health, abundance, and the ability to bear children.

But over time, that view shifted. Just like food was pulled into a hierarchy of "civilized" versus "uncivilized," bodies were too. In colonial America, Puritan and Protestant values reshaped how we viewed bodies. Larger bodies became linked to gluttony and a lack of self-control, and thinness was tied to purity, discipline, and moral virtue.

In *Fearing the Black Body*, sociologist Sabrina Strings traces how anti-fat bias was built over centuries, shaped first by Protestant ideas about self-control and moral virtue and later by racism. With the rise of the transatlantic slave trade, elite European thinkers began to tie fatness—especially on Black women's bodies—to "savagery," moral weakness, and racial inferiority. These ideas helped justify the dehumanization of Black people and uphold slavery. Thinness, meanwhile, became a way for white women to signal discipline, moral virtue, and racial superiority.

And as you saw in the previous chapter, these ideas shaped more than beauty standards. They shaped medicine, nutrition science, and the health guidelines that still affect our healthcare system today.

Scientific Racism and Medicine

As medicine and science advanced, these racist beliefs didn't disappear—they just became more "legitimized." Researchers twisted biology to argue that some races were biologically superior to others. White bodies became the "ideal," the gold standard every other body was measured against.

And doctors didn't just go along with this. They helped to reinforce it and taught it to others. Medical schools presented race as if it were a biological fact, when in reality race is something humans created, a way to group people by appearance and rank them. Black bodies were labeled "different," often described as stronger, less sensitive to pain, or built to endure more suffering. Some doctors even claimed Black skin was "thicker" or that Black people had different nervous systems. These myths justified giving less pain relief or offering less aggressive treatment, and they were written into medical textbooks for generations.

We can see how these dehumanizing beliefs still influence our medical system today. If you've ever had your child's growth chart compared to a "standard" curve without anyone asking about your family's genetics or felt dismissed at a doctor's visit because of weight, you've felt the ripple effects of this history.

When health systems are built on biased assumptions, they don't just ignore entire communities; they cause harm. And parents are often left trying to meet expectations that were never designed for their families in the first place.

Parent Reflection

Every one of us has inherited messages about food and bodies, messages that were shaped by systems that were never designed with our well-being in mind. We learned to distrust our hunger, to chase thinness, and to treat health as a measure of morality.

And now we're raising kids in a world that still pushes those same messages, sometimes louder than ever. Body shame doesn't just harm kids in larger bodies, it can hurt kids who are naturally thin, too, leaving them worried about "eating enough" or feeling like their bodies are wrong if they don't grow the way others expect.

This chapter isn't about calling you out. It's about calling you in, into awareness, healing, and a different kind of legacy. Once you can name the story you've been handed, you get to decide what to do with it, whether to keep passing it down or rewrite it into something more compassionate, inclusive, and free.

Weight Stigma: A Bigger Health Threat Than Weight Itself

As parents, we want the best for our kids. Yet in a culture shaped by racist and scientifically flawed ideas about body size, we've been told that the biggest threat to their health is the "childhood obesity epidemic." So it's no wonder many of us feel pressure to keep our kids "in a healthy weight range" or encourage them to "watch what they eat." It seems like the responsible thing to do.

But these cultural beliefs aren't simply prejudiced—they're actively harming our health. Let's explore how weight stigma and repeated attempts at dieting (often called "yo-yo dieting" or "weight cycling") lead to poor health outcomes and why protecting our kids from these issues is an important part of breaking the cycle of food and body shame.

Whether it's "fat" jokes on children's television (Peppa Pig, anyone?) or a medical professional who brushes off an individual's health concerns with advice to "just lose weight," weight stigma harms. And the judgment, teasing, and shame kids experience about their bodies is far more dangerous to their health than weight itself. Research links weight stigma to:

- **Low self-esteem:** Kids who experience weight stigma internalize negative messages, leading to poor self-image and a sense of worthlessness.
- **Lower academic performance:** Stigma and bullying can interfere with concentration, participation, and self-confidence in school. Some research even suggests that teachers may grade students in larger bodies more harshly.
- **Increased risk of bullying:** Children in larger bodies are more likely to be targeted for bullying, both by peers and, disturbingly, sometimes by adults.
- **Anxiety and depression:** There's a strong link between weight-based bullying and increased rates of anxiety, depression, and even suicidal thoughts or behaviors.
- **Increased risk of body dissatisfaction and disordered eating:** Weight stigma is associated with behaviors like binge eating, secretive eating, food restriction, and chronic dieting, even in young kids.

■ **Higher risk of eating disorders:** Contrary to what many people believe, weight-based teasing is one of the strongest predictors of developing an eating disorder, across all body sizes.

And this doesn't end in childhood. As kids grow into adults, weight stigma keeps taking a toll, often in deeper, more systemic ways. Living with constant judgment raises stress hormones like cortisol, which over time can increase the risk for health issues like heart disease, diabetes, and even some autoimmune conditions.

Many adults in larger bodies avoid going to the doctor because of past shame, or they get misdiagnosed when their concerns are blamed on weight instead of investigated fully. And the psychological effects of weight stigma in childhood linger. Disordered eating, low motivation to exercise, anxiety, depression, and low self-worth are all more common in adults who grew up facing weight stigma.

Yo-Yo Dieting: The Cycle That Makes Everything Worse

Most parents worry that if they don't help their kids "get healthy" now, they'll struggle with their weight forever. That's why programs like the Weight Watchers' Kurbo app for kids initially seemed appealing (thankfully, it was removed from the market in 2022).

But dieting doesn't prevent weight struggles. In fact, research shows it often predicts them. Rather than solving the problem, repeated dieting tends to backfire. The weight rarely stays off for long and over time, the cycle of losing and regaining weight (known as "weight cycling") disrupts metabolism, reduces muscle mass, and increases inflammation. These changes worsen the very conditions so often blamed on body size. Research also shows that most people who diet end up regaining more weight than they initially lost, leaving them at even higher weights in the long run.

This cycle not only puts stress on the body but also erodes trust in our hunger and fullness cues, making it harder to maintain consistent, supportive health behaviors like regular eating, joyful movement, or adequate rest. Dieting also increases our preoccupation with food and our bodies, and it's the single most common behavior that contributes to the development of an eating disorder.

Eating Disorders: More Common (and More Ignored) Than We Realize

When we think about raising healthy kids, most of us picture feeding them nutritious meals, keeping them active, and helping them feel confident. But there's something just as important and we don't talk about it nearly enough: eating disorders.

Here's what we wish more parents knew: Eating disorders are mental health conditions, and they're a lot more common than most of us realize. They're also the second deadliest mental illness after opioid addiction.

We can think of eating behaviors as a spectrum. On one end are people who reliably nourish their bodies. On the other are those with diagnosed eating disorders. And somewhere in the middle is where most people who live with disordered eating are—as many as 22% of children and up to 85% of adult women.

Eating Behaviors as a Spectrum

An eating disorder is a serious mental health condition marked by ongoing disruptions in eating behaviors along with distressing thoughts and emotions about food, body image, and weight. They often involve extreme restriction, loss of control around food, or intense fear of weight gain and significantly interfere with daily life. Eating disorders meet specific clinical criteria and typically require professional treatment.

Unfortunately, eating disorders are on the rise. Research shows that by young adulthood, as many as 1 in 5 girls (17.9%) and 1 in 40 boys (2.4%) will be diagnosed with an eating disorder. And these numbers don't even include all the kids quietly struggling without a diagnosis.

Disordered eating, on the other hand, is a general term for a range of harmful eating behaviors that don't meet the full criteria for an eating disorder but still negatively affect health and well-being. This can look like:

- Chronic dieting or skipping meals
- Rigid food rules ("I can never eat sugar")
- Emotional eating
- Frequent guilt or shame about food

Even though disordered eating isn't considered a mental illness, it is distressing, and it's one of the biggest risk factors for developing an eating disorder later. We aim to help you prevent your child from experiencing either.

Why So Many Eating Disorders Go Unnoticed

Eating disorders often fly under the radar, not because they're rare but because we've been conditioned to see them only when they show up in certain bodies.

When we think of eating disorders, most of us picture someone extremely thin, probably white, probably female. But the truth is, any child—any gender, any size, any race—can develop an eating disorder.

So why are so many cases underdiagnosed or overlooked?

- **Weight bias in healthcare:** Doctors often only screen thin kids for eating disorders. Larger-bodied kids might be praised for behaviors that are actually harmful, like skipping meals or over-exercising, because any weight loss is seen as "good."
- **Stereotypes:** If a child isn't visibly losing weight, people might assume they're "fine." But you can't tell if someone is struggling just by looking at them. Kids in all body sizes suffer, and their pain is real.

- **Cultural silence:** In many communities, especially those already facing stigma, mental health just isn't talked about openly. That means fewer diagnoses, less support, and more kids suffering in silence.
- **Access to care:** Eating disorder treatment is hard to access, especially in under-resourced or rural areas. Without the right providers, many families are left without answers or help.

To complicate things further, many people live with disordered eating for years without a formal diagnosis, but their quality of life still suffers.

The Stereotypes Hurt

Despite the common stereotype that eating disorders typically affect young, white girls, eating disorders affect people of every race, gender, and body size. In fact, research reveals patterns that directly contradict the stereotype:

- Black, Latinx, and Asian Americans are actually more likely to engage in disordered eating, and teens who face racial discrimination are three times more likely to develop binge eating disorder.
- About 4% of males have had a diagnosed eating disorder, and rates in men are now rising even faster than they are for women.
- As many as 40% of children in the "overweight" or "obese" BMI categories show signs of disordered eating.
- People with BMIs over 30 are more than twice as likely to struggle with disordered eating yet only half as likely to be diagnosed compared to those in the "underweight" or "normal weight" categories.

These stereotypes are especially harmful because when children of color or those in larger bodies restrict food or overexercise, their behaviors are too often ignored or even praised as "healthy habits," leaving vulnerable kids at greater risk of untreated eating disorders.

EXPERT INSIGHT: Higher Risk, Lower Support: Eating Disorders in Communities of Color

Dr. Whitney Trotter DNP, PMHNP-BC, RDN, @whitneytrotter.rd

Communities of color often face a deep injustice when it comes to eating disorders: higher risk and burden yet lower visibility and access to care. Prior to 2020 you rarely saw people of color being represented in media, advertisement, clinical roles, or research in the field of eating disorders. Stigma, cultural stereotypes, and systemic racism often mean disordered eating is overlooked or misdiagnosed, leaving individuals without the support they need. At the same time, structural barriers like lack of insurance coverage, culturally competent providers, and treatment affordability widen the care gap. The result is a cycle where suffering is both amplified and silenced—a reality we must work to dismantle.

The Role of Trauma, Sensory Needs, and Mental Health

Not every eating disorder comes from wanting a smaller body. Some kids struggle with food intake related to anxiety, depression, sensory challenges, or past food trauma, and diet culture only makes it worse.

A child with Avoidant/Restrictive Food Intake Disorder (ARFID) might fear being judged for preferring chicken nuggets and fries, even though that's all they can manage to eat. A teen with irritable bowel syndrome (IBS) might avoid eating because of stomach pain and be praised for losing weight. None of this is healthy.

And for kids who've experienced adverse childhood experiences (ACEs), food often becomes a way to cope with stress or fear. That can lead to binge eating, restricting, or unpredictable eating patterns that are hard to change, especially when they experience shame for these very behaviors.

Fortunately, there are steps we can take to protect our kids from suffering from this spectrum of food harms.

The AAP's Three Red Flags

In a 2016 clinical report titled "Preventing Obesity and Eating Disorders in Adolescents," the American Academy of Pediatrics (AAP) highlighted three big risk factors for eating disorders in teens:

- **Dieting:** Any restriction of food—either by the child or adult-led—with the goal of weight loss
- **Weight talk:** Comments about your own weight or your child's weight
- **Weight teasing:** Hurtful jokes or remarks about body size from family, peers, or even teachers

And did you catch the title of that paper? The same factors that help prevent eating disorders—avoiding dieting, weight talk, and weight teasing—also protect kids from harmful patterns linked to weight gain, like yo-yo dieting, binge eating, and weight stigma. These patterns contribute significantly to both physical and emotional health risks, regardless of a child's size.

Bringing It Home

This chapter was a lot. You've just traced how body ideals shifted from celebration to shame, how those ideas were tied to racism and morality, and how they're still shaping healthcare, nutrition advice, and the messages our kids hear today.

If you're feeling emotional after reading this, please know you're not the only one. But awareness is power. Noticing how weight stigma and diet culture show up at the doctor's office, at school, in the media, and even in our self-talk gives us a chance to respond differently.

We can teach our kids that health is about how they feel in their bodies, not what their bodies look like. We can create homes where no one feels ashamed of their size, where food is about nourishment and joy, not punishment or control, and where kids aren't pushed into harmful eating patterns just to fit in.

One Simple Step

The next time you catch yourself linking your child's body size to their health, pause and ask: Is this fact, or is this diet culture talking? Would I be thinking the same if my child were a different size? Reminding yourself that health cannot be measured by size alone helps you respond with curiosity and care instead of worry.

Your Food Positivity Practice

Choosing New Body Rules: *Growing Beyond What No Longer Serves Us*

4

You're the Narrator Now: Turning Awareness into Action

At a barbecue recently, my daughter filled her plate with chips and hot dogs. I felt my stomach twist, remembering how my cousins once teased me for "eating like a pig." I so desperately wanted to stop her, but I managed to let her be. She sat with the other kids, laughing and fitting right in. I felt so grateful that she could just be a kid, but it also hurt to realize how I should have had that experience, too.

—Shelby

IF YOU'VE MADE it this far, pause for a moment. What you're doing right now is brave. You've opened yourself up to rethinking the messages you were given about health, food, and bodies, and that takes courage.

You might be feeling a mix of emotions right now such as guilt, sadness, or maybe even anger. You might be remembering the food rules you grew up with, remembering the comments adults made about your body, or noticing how easily we absorb beliefs from family, culture, and media without ever choosing them.

That's not failure; that's awareness. And awareness is the first step toward change.

And still, even with that awareness, you might be thinking: "I still kinda wish my body looked different" or "I just don't want my kid to struggle the way I did."

Those feelings are valid. Wanting to be accepted, to fit in, to protect your child from harm. That's not vanity; that's being human. So much of what we've been taught about food and bodies is tied to our deep need to belong.

Let's reflect on what we've been carrying and start to set it down. You'll see why this work matters, not just for you but for the legacy you're creating, and you'll leave ready to turn the page into Part II, where we shift our focus to the kids we're raising and how to give them something better.

Belonging vs. Fitting In

So much of what we've been taught about food and bodies is really about our deep need to belong—to feel accepted, to fit in, to be safe in our communities.

> "Fitting in is about assessing a situation and becoming who you need to be to be accepted. Belonging, on the other hand, doesn't require us to change who we are; it requires us to be who we are."
>
> —Brené Brown, *The Gifts of Imperfection*

When we start to see how much of diet culture is about fitting in, following rules, shrinking ourselves, and earning approval, it makes sense why letting go of those rules can feel so scary. Belonging asks something different. It invites us and our kids to come to the table as our full selves, without changing to meet someone else's standard. And when we choose belonging over fitting in, we not only free ourselves from the pressure to perform, we create a home where our kids feel safe to do the same.

Two Things Can Be True

You can be ready to challenge diet culture *and* still carry old beliefs about food and bodies.

You can want to raise body-confident kids *and* still struggle with your own reflection in the mirror.

You can dream of a better world *and* still feel unsure how to talk about dessert.

This doesn't mean you're doing it wrong; it means you're unlearning and learning. And what matters most is what you choose to do next, because that's what shapes the story your child will carry forward.

Looking Back, Moving Forward

"Rather than staying stuck in shame or denial, we need to now reckon with all the expectations we've absorbed—and figure out how to begin the process of letting them go."

—Virginia Sole-Smith, *Fat Talk*

Throughout Part I, we've explored how our understanding of health has been shaped by systems that were never designed to support us. We've unpacked how diet culture shows up in our food systems, how we measure health, and even where many of our parenting norms came from. We've traced the historical roots of diet culture and seen how racism, classism, and religious morality shaped what foods are labeled "good," what bodies are considered "healthy," and who gets blamed when health outcomes don't match a narrow ideal.

And we've looked inward, starting to name the food and body rules we carry, often quietly and unconsciously, into our parenting. That's big. That's brave. That matters.

What We've Been Told Isn't the Whole Truth

For generations, we've been taught that health is a personal responsibility and weight is the ultimate marker of health—that if our kids eat the "right" things and grow the "right" way, we're succeeding, and if not, we've somehow failed.

But we now know this isn't the whole story. Health is shaped far more by social determinants—things like access to food, housing, healthcare, and community support—than by what's on our plates.

Food and body rules weren't designed to help families thrive. They're tools used to control us, and they are deeply rooted in systems of power and oppression.

That history didn't stay in the past. It's still with us and lives on in modern wellness culture, in anti-fat bias, in how we label food as "good" or "bad," and in what our kids pick up and absorb from the world around them.

And here's the thing: even when we *know* better, it can still be hard to *do* it differently. Because diet culture is sneaky. It shows up in "just one more bite," in "you've had enough," in praising smaller bodies, and in fearing weight gain, even in children.

But once you *see* it, you can start to shift it.

Food Positivity Starts Here

Food Positivity isn't about throwing nutrition out the window. We're not pretending that all foods offer the same nutrients or that we eat different foods for the same reason. That's like saying microwaving Tuesday night mac and cheese and decorating Christmas cookies are the same—one is about getting through the day, the other is about making a memory. Both matter. Both have a place in a healthy relationship with food. Food Positivity helps kids (and us!) see that all of it belongs—the quick dinners, the comfort foods, the balanced meals, the holiday favorites—without guilt or shame.

It's about becoming your child's trusted guide, their food leader. It's about creating a space that supports the whole child physically, emotionally, and socially where children (and parents, too!) can feel safe, valued, and confident around food. It's about more than just *what* food we serve; it's about *how* we offer it, talk about it, and experience it together.

When kids experience food with safety, trust, and joy, they grow into adults who can make choices that truly support them. They will be adults who might decide on a veggie and egg scramble instead of a muffin before a long morning meeting not because it's "healthier" but because they know how to tune in to their body cues and honor their needs.

Food Positivity is about raising healthy kids from the inside out. It's about helping them eat a variety of foods, feel connected at the table, and learn to listen to their bodies. And maybe just as important? It's about freeing *you* from the guilt and anxiety you've been carrying too.

This is the heart of this book.

You're the Narrator Now

By now, you've seen how deeply diet culture has shaped our food systems, our health standards, and even the way we think about bodies. You've traced how those messages were passed down from generation to generation, and you've started to notice which ones still live in your own self-talk today.

And now it's your turn to write the story.

Language isn't neutral, and neither is silence. Every comment, every sigh at the dinner table, every offhand remark about your body or your child's body teaches something. Our words teach kids what to believe about food, self-worth, and belonging.

For many of us, the scripts we were handed were rooted in shame and fear. We were taught to shrink, restrict, earn, or hide. But we can choose different words. We can offer the voice that will become our children's inner voice, one rooted in curiosity, respect, and trust. That shift doesn't just change what happens at mealtimes; it changes the kind of home our children grow up in. A home where food isn't feared, bodies aren't judged, and everyone feels like they belong.

And if you ever feel doubt creeping in or catch yourself slipping back into old scripts, pause for a moment. Take a breath. And come back to this truth:

You are not behind.

You're not too late.

You're not broken.

The fact that you're here—reading, reflecting, trying—is enough.

You are enough. You are exactly the parent your child needs.

Bringing It Home

There's no right or wrong. No one "best" way. No one-size-fits-all. No perfect. No all-or-nothing. All you need is to be willing to learn, unlearn, reconnect, and keep showing up.

It might look like dropping the "clean plate" rule.

Or enjoying dessert together a few more nights a week.

Or pausing before praising someone's weight loss (or a child's naturally thin body).

Or simply choosing to say nothing about someone's body at all.

Start today with one thought, one phrase, one moment, or one meal. These small shifts may be quiet, but they're life-changing, and you've already begun.

And now, as we move into Part II, we'll shift the focus from the systems that shaped us to the kids we're raising today, exploring how to meet them where they are, build trust and confidence, and become the parent you wish you'd had.

One Simple Step

Notice one food or body rule you've been carrying, such as "clean your plate" or "dessert only on weekends," or a comment you catch yourself thinking about your body.

Pause and ask, "Do I actually believe this? Does it support the kind of relationship with food I want for my kids?"

If the answer is no, try letting that rule go just once. See how it feels.

Your Food Positivity Practice

Creating Our Family's Food & Body Culture: *Choosing What Belongs in Our Story*

PART

Whole-Child Development and What Kids Are Learning About Food and Bodies

5

Nutrition Matters: It Starts with Positive Feeding Foundations

I put so much effort into making healthy meals for my family. My son used to eat what I made, but lately dinner has been so frustrating. He'll sometimes eat the bread or pasta, but when I tell him to take a few bites of vegetables too, he often lashes out at me! Last night he said he wasn't hungry and wanted to leave the table, but a few minutes later he was asking for dessert. I told him if he's not hungry enough to eat the healthy food I made, he's not hungry enough for dessert either. I worry constantly that he's not getting the nutrients he needs, but I don't know how to get him to eat healthy food without a fight.

—Jasmine

LET'S SAY IT again: Nutrition *absolutely* matters.

If you're anything like us, you've probably had moments where you wished there was a simple way to "get" your child to eat well. Maybe you've Googled "picky eating tips" at 11 p.m. or worried that cereal-for-dinner nights mean you're doing something wrong. (You're not doing it wrong.) You're human and so is your kiddo.

But most advice about feeding kids is as outdated as the one-size-fits-all version of the "healthy plate." From hiding veggies to pressuring with "just one bite" or "no dessert until you finish your dinner" to relying on "they'll eat when they're hungry," these strategies often backfire. Even well-meaning tips—like focusing on what foods do in the body or praising kids for what they eat—can actually make mealtimes more stressful and do little to help kids feel more confident around food.

You know by now that health is about so much more than what's on our plates, and nutrition is just one piece of the puzzle. As pediatric dietitians (and moms), we care deeply about what kids eat—and just as much about how we offer and teach them about food.

That's why we believe our job is much bigger than *"just* nutrition." We want to raise kids who trust their bodies, enjoy a wide variety of foods, and feel confident making choices long after they've left our kitchen tables. That's why we're starting with understanding your child's world—their brain, body, beliefs, and needs—so you can truly see the whole child sitting at your table.

This chapter will give you a new kind of roadmap, one rooted in trust, stability, and respect for your child's individual needs. You'll discover the foundations kids need to build a positive relationship with food from the inside out: support for their physical growth, emotional safety, and body trust.

Because *what* you feed matters, but *how* your child feels at the table matters even more.

Your Role: The Food Leader

Truly supporting nutrition means stepping into a different kind of leadership role and being the steady guide your child can count on. In Part III, we'll dig deeper into just how to do this with practical, doable strategies that help you lead with confidence and feed with compassion.

For now, while we're focused on understanding your child's experience and needs, here's what you need to know.

Just like guiding your child through a predictable bedtime routine, your job is to take the lead at mealtimes. That means planning and preparing meals, deciding when and where food is offered based on your child's needs, and making sure a mix of nourishing (and yes, delicious!) foods show up alongside their safe favorites. Some nights, that might look like adding a comfort food after a rough day, sitting quietly with them as they decide what to eat, or trusting them to stop when they're full. The most important thing to remember is this: **Food only becomes nutrition when your child actually eats it**.

And a balanced plate doesn't mean much if your child doesn't feel safe, supported, and ready to eat. That's why before we talk about *what* to feed kids, we need to first focus on *how* we feed them. The mood, the energy in the room, and whether your child feels safe showing up to the table exactly as they are, is the very first step.

And that's where the **Food Positivity Foundations** come in.

Parent Reflection

As you read this chapter with your own child in mind, we hope you'll also reflect on everything we unpacked in Part I and consider how those issues shape a person's ability to truly nourish themselves. Whether it's growing up in a food-insecure home, hearing that your family's cultural foods are "unhealthy," or being taught that body size matters more than genuine nourishment, each of these experiences stem from the same root problem: a lack of the fundamental supports we all need to thrive.

You may also find yourself thinking about your own childhood and what could have been different about your relationship with food and your body if you'd grown up in a home that fostered these needs. While we can't change the past, what matters now is how you choose to move forward with your child.

Building Your Framework Foundations

Food Positivity is about supporting your whole child—body, mind, and spirit. If we want kids to learn how to nourish their bodies, not out of guilt, pressure, or blind obedience, but because it feels good to connect with their bodies and care for themselves, we need a new perspective. True support for whole-child well-being means considering *two perspectives*—the child's and the adult's.

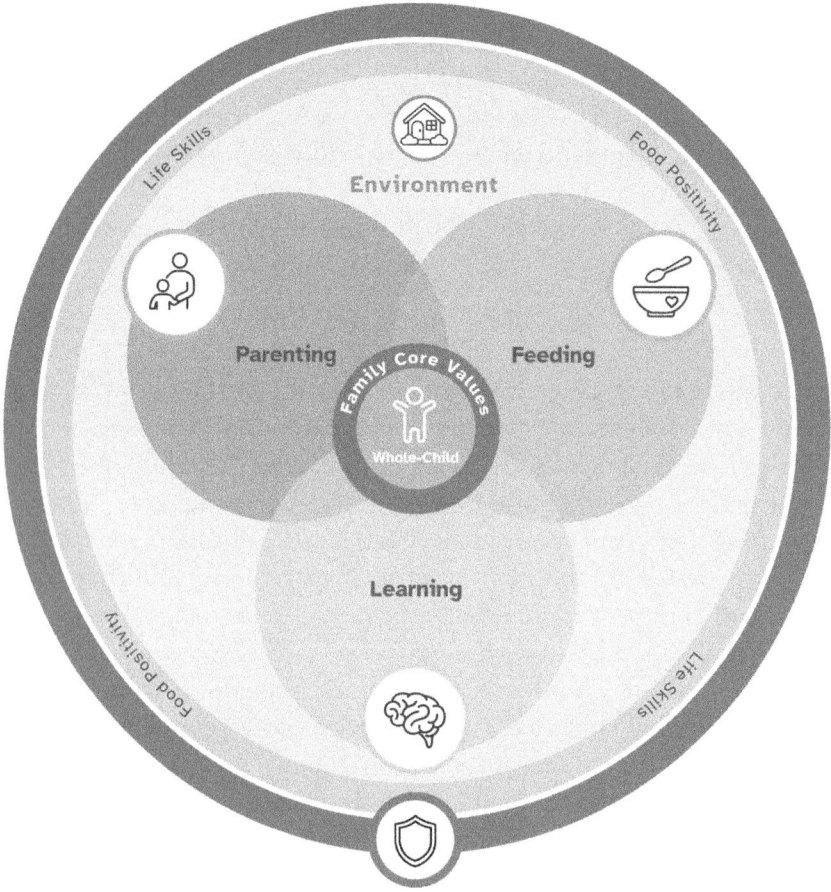

We build this understanding layer by layer through your four Food Positivity Foundations that form your **Food Positivity Framework**. The four foundations offer practical tools for all aspects of food and body learning, and we simplify them here by how they show up in daily life: **Feeding, Environment, Learning,** and **Parenting**. Within each of these foundations, the layers remain the same but shift based on perspective.

What's a Framework, Anyway?

A framework is just a way to take big, messy ideas and organize them into something you can actually use. Think of it like the frame of a house; it gives structure and support, but you still arrange the furniture inside in a way that works for your family.

You might have heard of frameworks like *Intuitive Eating*, *Montessori*, or *Conscious Parenting*. They're not step-by-step plans but guiding principles people can lean on to work toward a desired result.

The Food Positivity Framework works the same way. It's not a rigid checklist. It's a set of guiding ideas you can return to as you raise kids in a world full of food fears and body pressures. And because most of us weren't taught these skills growing up, this framework gives you something steady to lean on as you support your kids and yourself in building a lasting, positive relationship with food and their bodies.

Let's look at the pieces that make up every Food Positivity Foundation.

The Whole-Child

At the center of each Food Positivity Foundation is the Whole-Child, not just their eating habits, but their growing brain, emotions, senses, identity, and lived experiences. A child who needs help calming big feelings also needs that same sense of safety when deciding whether to try a new food. Body trust, autonomy, emotional safety, and belonging don't magically pause at the table; they're part of how kids learn everything, including how to feel about food and their bodies. Emotional safety is what lets kids exhale, knowing they won't be shamed, pressured, or criticized so they can relax and focus on connection and learning.

Family Core Values

The first layer is always about your Family Core Values, your "compass." There's no one-size-fits-all or "right" set of values, but when kids consistently hear clear, supportive messages at home, those messages become the steady foundation your child grows on. (You'll learn how to define and live out your Family Core Values in Chapter 10.)

Needs and Skills

Within each foundation, following the Whole-Child and Family Core Values, there are two complementary layers that work together to help you meet your child's deepest needs, guide their growth, and raise kids who feel safe, capable, and free from food and body shame: Needs and Skills.

Each layer has two perspectives: yours and your child's.

Kids do the *growing*. Parents do the *guiding*. These two perspectives work together to meet needs and build skills they'll carry for life.

Here's a simple way to see how these layers work together:

	Needs *What Kids Need*	Skills *What Kids Practice and Learn*
Growing (child)	**Growing Needs:** What kids need most to feel safe, supported, and ready to learn.	**Growing Skills:** What kids are learning to do: making choices, noticing body cues, exploring with curiosity, and finding where they belong.
Guiding (parent)	**Guiding Needs:** What parents need to show up calm, grounded, and ready to meet their child's needs.	**Guiding Skills:** What parents practice to create the conditions for growth: modeling, guiding, and honoring their child's efforts.

Growing Needs = What Kids Need First

Before kids can explore food with curiosity, build confidence in their bodies, or develop new skills, their most basic emotional needs must be met. These Growing Needs—feeling safe, supported, and able to trust themselves—are the foundation for a positive relationship with food and body. When kids feel secure, connected, and respected, they're more likely to show up fully at meals, in the kitchen, and in the world around them.

These needs change as kids grow and even shift from day to day. Some days your child may seem calm and confident; other days they may need extra reassurance. What matters most is your steady presence and care. Little things, like staying calm when they're overwhelmed, keeping mealtimes pressure-free, or respecting their cues, send a powerful message over time. When their needs are met often enough, your child can relax, stay curious, and engage with food in ways that help them grow.

Later, we'll explore your role with Guiding Needs (Chapter 11) and Guiding Skills (Chapter 9). But first, let's look more closely at your child's perspective. Their Growing Needs show up every day at the table, shaping how they experience food, their body, and their connection with you.

Growing Skills = What Kids Are Learning to Do

Now that we've looked at your child's Needs in the Feeding Foundation, let's step back and see how those Needs connect to the next layer of the Framework—the Growing Skills that build on them.

Once their needs are met, kids are ready to practice Growing Skills: the abilities that help them make choices, notice and respond to their body cues, explore with curiosity, and feel like they belong.

These skills grow through hands-on experiences and everyday moments, with lots of starts, stops, and do-overs along the way. They don't develop all at once or in a straight line. Some kids jump ahead in one area while needing extra support in another. Growth looks different for every child, and leaps, pauses, and backslides are all part of the process.

Your job isn't to force progress or growth. It's to create safe, supportive chances to practice. With patience, curiosity, and care, you help strengthen these skills until they start to feel natural for your child.

The Food Positivity Feeding Foundations

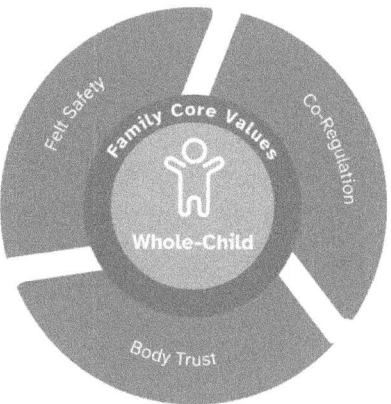

We're starting with Feeding because it's where all of these layers show up most clearly in everyday life. The Feeding Foundations focus on the social and emotional climate around food and the daily conditions that shape how kids feel about eating, their bodies, and themselves.

It's not about what's on the plate. It's about how your child experiences the meal: Do they feel safe? Do they feel heard? Do they feel free to explore and connect? When we understand their Growing Needs in this context, we can support them in building trust, curiosity, and a positive relationship with food that lasts.

You've Been Laying the Foundation All Along

Think back to those first days of starting solids. Maybe your baby grinned as they smeared avocado across the highchair tray or giggled after a big slurp of yogurt while you laughed along. That messy, playful exploration? That was Felt Safety. That was Co-Regulation. That was Body Trust developing right in front of you.

Many of these foundations were already present in the early feeding relationship, especially if you followed your baby's cues and offered food without pressure. But over time, things can shift.

Developmental changes (like toddlers craving independence), outside influences (like diet culture creeping into daycare), and even the sheer exhaustion of day-to-day parenting can chip away at that foundation. Suddenly, mealtimes can feel more like a power struggle than a playful connection.

That doesn't mean you've done anything wrong; it just means it's time to reconnect with what matters most. It is time to rebuild trust, nurture regulation, and meet your child right where they are. And you've already started just by reading this. You're showing up with intention, and that's the first step toward a calmer, more connected table.

Feeding Foundations: Growing Needs (Felt Safety, Co-Regulation, Body Trust)

Let's start by focusing on your child's three key Growing Needs: Felt Safety, Co-Regulation, and Body Trust. These Growing Needs make everything else possible and lay the groundwork for curiosity, confidence, and connection at the table.

Felt Safety (Growing Need)

Safety makes everything else possible.

Felt Safety isn't just knowing you're safe; it's *feeling* safe deep in your body. For kids, that means way more than hearing "you're okay" from a grown-up (even though *you* may know that they're objectively safe). It means actually *believing* it in their nervous system. You can often see it when their shoulders drop, their breathing slows, and their face softens. Their brain and body get the message: *I can settle, I'm safe here.*

When that sense of safety is missing, our bodies move into protection mode: fight, flight, or freeze. What looks like big feelings, food obsessions, "picky" eating, or outright food refusal isn't bad behavior; it's a nervous system doing its job. And those protection responses aren't just triggered by major stress. It can be something small, like a loud noise at the table, a new food that feels too unfamiliar, a long day at school, or the stress they sense in *your* body when you're worried they're not eating enough. Kids pick up on it all.

When kids feel safe and can settle, everything shifts. Their curiosity kicks in, their appetites open up, and their brain is ready to learn and explore. You might notice they stay at the table longer, play with their food, or show little sparks of flexibility—signs that their body feels safe enough to stay connected.

> "When the quality of the eating experience improves for the child, the quantity and variety can then improve, but at the child's pace"
>
> —Katja Rowell, *Love Me, Feed Me*

Everyday Moments That Support Felt Safety

- Trusting they won't be pushed to taste something they're not ready for
- Saying "no" and having that "no" respected
- Feeling confident their caregiver will be present and supportive no matter what

---

For Families Navigating More

For some families, building Felt Safety takes extra care, and that's okay. If your child has experienced food insecurity or trauma or is neurodivergent, you may need to go slower. That might look like making sure they know exactly when the next meal is coming, honoring their safe foods more consistently, or working with a feeding specialist. Progress may look different or take longer, but the same foundations of Felt Safety, Co-Regulation, and Body Trust still apply.

We'll share more strategies for supporting neurodivergent eaters and kids with feeding challenges in Chapter 13, but for now, keep this in mind: what matters most is meeting your child where they are, not where someone else says they should be.

Co-Regulation (Growing Need)

Connection helps kids return to calm.

Co-Regulation is about guiding your child through big feelings by staying calm, present, and connected while they learn to do the same. It's not about fixing their emotions or preventing every mealtime meltdown—it's about helping them find their way back to that safe, settled place. And Co-Regulation isn't something you explain; it's something your child *feels*. Their brain and body get the message: *I'm not alone. I can find my way back to calm with you beside me.*

If you've been at the table with a tired, hungry, or overwhelmed kid, you know how quickly emotions can take over. A new food can feel scary. A missed snack can turn into a hangry meltdown. A bright light, loud sound, or strong smell can throw their nervous system into overdrive. What looks like "bad behavior" is often just a body asking for help.

When kids feel your calm beside them, everything shifts. Instead of needing you to fix their feelings, they borrow your steady presence to ride the wave and start making sense of their feelings. Over time, these repeated moments teach them that their feelings are valid, that they can work through them, and find their way back to calm. This helps build their inner roadmap for self-regulation—how to trust themselves, how to stay connected, and how to feel safe and cared for around food.

Co-Regulation as a Cycle Breaker

If no one modeled a calm, steady presence for you as a child, it makes sense that doing the same for your child now feels hard, maybe even impossible. Your body learned survival, not safety. And that's not your fault.

Still, as your child's grown-up, you have the chance to break the cycle. Start small, like softening your voice or taking a breath before reacting. (We'll share even more strategies in Chapter 10.) And when you lose it (because we all do), reconnect with care. You're doing the work your younger self deserved and your child will benefit from every step you take.

Everyday Moments That Support Co-Regulation

- Hearing you describe their experiences and reactions without judgment
- Experiencing big feelings or sensations and working through them with your support
- Feeling comforted when their calm, trusted adult is simply nearby

Body Trust (Growing Need)

Trust grows when kids believe their body is worth listening to.

Bonus Handout via the QR Code: Building Body Trust: A Parent's Quick-Start Guide

Body Trust is the deep, internal knowing that your body is good, wise, and capable of telling you what it needs. Kids build that trust through small, everyday moments when they listen, honor their needs, and stay connected to what their body is telling them. Their brain and body get the message: *What I feel matters. My body is telling me something important. I can listen and respond.*

Kids are born with Body Trust. Babies cry when they're hungry, turn away when they're full, or look for closeness when they need comfort. But over time, that natural wisdom can get interrupted. When kids are pressured with the "three-bite rule," praised for cleaning their plate, or told they're "done" when they still feel hungry, they start to wonder if their body's signals are wrong or if *they're* wrong for having them.

When kids feel free to follow their hunger, fullness, and sensory cues, everything shifts. They learn their body is wise, that their needs matter, and that grown-ups will listen. That trust eventually expands beyond food into movement, rest, boundaries, and speaking up for themselves. Each time you show your child that you trust their body, you strengthen the quiet voice inside them that says: *I can trust myself.*

Everyday Moments That Support Body Trust

- Eating without feeling pressured, bribed, or praised for how much they eat
- Hearing food and bodies talked about in neutral, nonjudgmental ways
- Exploring new foods when they feel ready, not on someone else's timeline

When Food Doesn't Feel Reliable

Body Trust is harder to build when food feels scarce. As we uncovered in Part I, experiences like food insecurity or repeated restriction can signal danger to a child's nervous system. Eating past fullness, hoarding, or fixating on foods aren't bad habits—they're protective responses from a body doing exactly what it's designed to do in the face of uncertainty. Regular, predictable access to food and a calm, consistent approach to feeding will help children—and adults—rebuild this trust over time.

Feeding Foundations: Growing Skills (Autonomy, Self-Regulation, Playful Exploration, Belonging + Identity)

Now let's bring Growing Skills back to the table. In the Feeding Foundations, kids practice four key skills: Autonomy, Self-Regulation, Playful Exploration, and Belonging + Identity. These skills aren't just about eating; they shape how kids see themselves, trust their bodies, and feel like they belong.

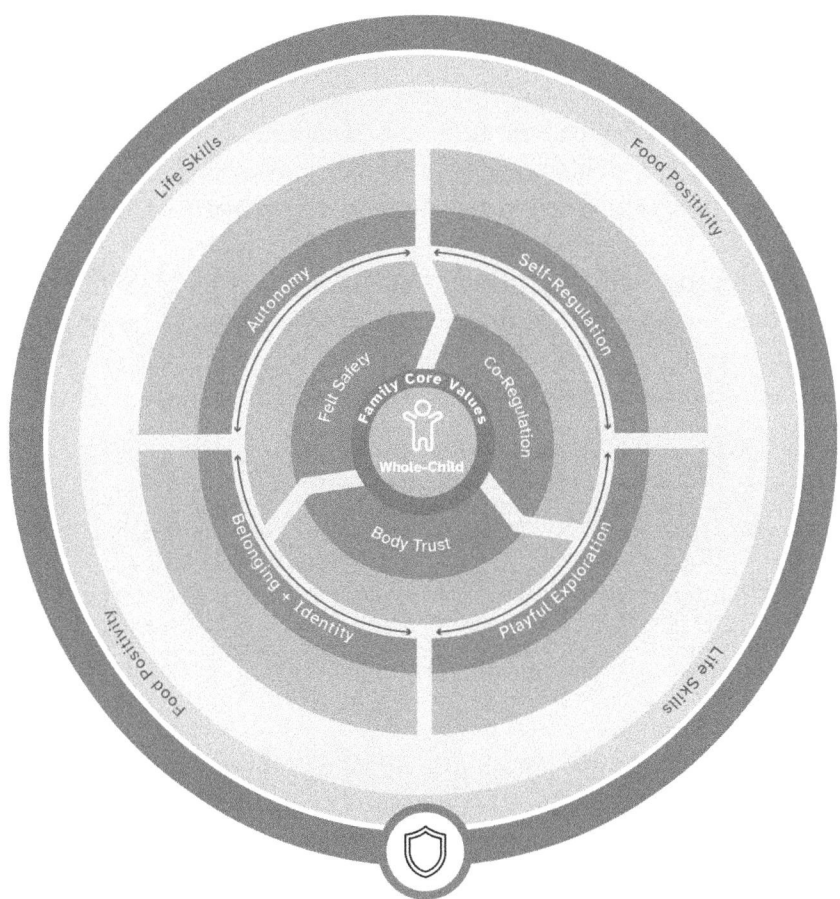

Autonomy (Growing Skill)

Confidence grows when kids know their choices matter.

Bonus Handout via the QR Code: What Autonomy Can Look Like at Every Age

Autonomy is your child learning, *I can do things for myself.* But it doesn't mean leaving them to figure it out alone. It's guided independence, giving them safe opportunities to make choices, express preferences, and take part in decisions about food, with you right there as their steady guide. Their brain and body get the message: My *choices matter. My voice matters. I can be part of this process.*

Kids are wired to seek independence, and if they don't have safe, supported ways to express it, they'll often fight for it. This can look like refusing food, pushing back at the table, or turning mealtime into a battle. That's not defiance; it's development.

When kids are given choices, like picking between two snacks or helping prep part of a meal, they feel respected, feel empowered, and are more open to trying new food. Over time, these moments build a sense of agency, the belief that what they do and say matters. And that belief grows into the confidence to speak up when they're hungry, uncomfortable, or feeling pressured.

Supporting Autonomy doesn't mean "anything goes." You're still the Food Leader—setting the rhythm, providing a variety of food, offering new foods for exposure, and holding boundaries with kindness and consistency (we'll look at just how to do this in Chapter 12).

Everyday Moments That Support Autonomy
- Choosing between two snack options you offer
- Deciding what order to eat the foods on their plate
- Helping in the kitchen by cooking, stirring, or setting the table

Self-Regulation (Growing Skill)

Kids thrive when they can tune in.

Self-Regulation is your child's growing ability to notice what is happening inside their body and respond in ways that help them feel calm, connected, and in control. It isn't about being calm all the time. It's about learning to pause, check in, and choose a helpful next step. It shows up at the table and everywhere else. Their brain and body get the message: *I can notice what I feel and choose what I do next.*

Tantrums over the "wrong" brand of chicken nuggets or endless snack requests aren't bad behavior. They're signs your child is still learning how to cope and communicate. Self-Regulation is how kids respond to the signals their body sends: hunger, fullness, frustration, boredom, or excitement. Learning to tune in and manage those cues takes time. The brain's self-management system, called *executive function*, is still "under construction" well into the teen years. When kids are hungry, tired, stressed, or overwhelmed by sensory input, that system can easily get thrown off. What may look like a meltdown is often your child asking for help in the only way their body knows how.

And when pressure, restriction, or shame enter the picture, the process gets harder. Phrases like "If you don't eat now, you're not getting anything later" or "You've had too much sugar today" may "work" in the moment, but over time they fuel power struggles, shrink variety, and chip away at Body Trust. (More on this in Chapter 9!)

Self-Regulation grows best in a steady, low-pressure environment where you model the skills you want to teach. With your calm presence, kids learn to pause before reacting, stay curious with new foods, and stop when they've had enough (even with dessert!). Over time, those small moments add up to the regulation skills they'll carry for life.

Everyday Moments That Support Self-Regulation
- Noticing when they feel full and stopping, even if there's food left
- Asking for a snack when they feel hungry, even if it's not mealtime
- Using a fidget toy, wiggle break, or softer lighting to stay settled at meals

---

Research Spotlight: Born for Self-Regulation

If you've spent years ignoring or second-guessing your own hunger cues, it may feel impossible to believe that anyone—let alone a child—can naturally know how much to eat. But research shows

(continued)

(*continued*)

that children truly can regulate their food intake when parents provide supportive conditions.

Studies from researchers including Leann Birch and Ellyn Satter have repeatedly shown that kids adjust how much they eat depending on how filling the food is. They also balance their food intake out across meals and days, generally getting the nutrition they need from what you serve. What gets in the way is when adults—or diet culture messages—interfere, teaching us to override our own cues, eat more or less than we truly want, or treat beloved foods as forbidden and highly desirable.

We encourage you to adopt a positive, open-minded approach to your child's Self-Regulation ability. Believe in them. . .they were born for this!

Playful Exploration (Growing Skill)

Curiosity is the gateway to learning.

Kids are natural explorers, and play is how they learn and make sense of the world, including food. Playful Exploration is pressure free food exposure. It gives kids the freedom to discover food on their own terms, with their senses, creativity, and imagination. Their brain and body get the message: *Food is fun and safe to explore. My curiosity is welcome here.*

As grown-ups, our goal is often "getting" kids to eat in ways that line up with our expectations: "put it in your mouth, chew 10 times, and then you can spit it out," "hurry up and eat," or "stop playing with your food." But when play and exploration—the very work of childhood—shifts from curiosity to pressure, or from self-discovery to pleasing an adult, kids often pull away and resist, and mealtime can turn into a battle.

That's because eating is just one part of the learning process and usually the very last step. Kids often need dozens of mini-experiments: smelling, sorting, dissecting, watching you eat it, asking questions, playing pretend, or even making a mess before they're ready to take a bite.

When we give kids the space to engage with food through play, they build comfort and confidence over time. You can see it in everyday moments—when a child squishes berries into "paint," asks how M&M's are made, picks basil from the garden, or lines up carrot sticks just to see which one is longest. Each of these small experiments tells them: *It's okay to go at my own pace. I get to decide when I'm ready to taste.*

Everyday Moments That Support Playful Exploration
- Exploring food with their senses before deciding to taste it
- Helping with meal prep without any pressure to eat what they make
- Watching others' enjoyment and learning before trying it themselves

"Play is really the work of childhood."

—Fred Rogers

Play Looks Different for Every Child

Some kids dive in headfirst, stacking, playing pretend, or licking everything in sight. Others take their time and observe quietly. Some less obvious ways that children explore food include:

- Poking food with the back of a spoon
- Watching a sibling try something new
- Asking questions about how a food is made
- Helping prepare the food, but choosing not to eat it

Whether they explore loudly or quietly, messily or carefully, their way of learning deserves our respect. And every safe, pressure-free interaction builds confidence, even if they don't take a single bite. More on this in Chapter 9 and Chapter 17.

Belonging + Identity (Growing Skill)

Belonging begins when kids feel safe to be themselves.

Belonging + Identity grows when children feel accepted as they are. At the table, that looks like having their food, body, and culture welcomed without judgment. When the signals around them are warm and affirming, kids learn that their differences are valued, not erased. Their brain and body get the message: *I'm welcome here. Who I am belongs.*

When belonging is missing, kids absorb harmful messages about identity and self-worth. At home, it might sound like food preferences being dismissed, a request met with a sigh, or a body being criticized. Outside the home, it might look like lunchboxes labeled "weird" or cultural foods called "junk." Over time, those signals pile up until a child begins to believe: *My food is wrong. My body doesn't fit in. I need to change myself to belong.*

But when kids feel accepted, everything shifts. They relax into being themselves, take pride in their culture, and grow confident not just in what they eat but in who they are.

Belonging grows at home when a child's "safe food" is served without judgment or when a grandparent's recipe is cooked with love. It grows outside the home when differences are celebrated—like at school, when someone asks, "What's this dish called in your language?" or when the class reads a story about different food traditions and invites kids to share their own. In those everyday moments, children feel seen and valued, learning that their preferences, culture, and body all matter.

Everyday Moments That Support Belonging and Identity
- Recognizing their sensory preferences as valid and not shameful
- Remembering there's no single "right" way to eat or grow
- Experiencing food-related religious or cultural practices

Food Positivity Life Skills = What Kids Carry for Life

When you nurture your child's Growing Needs and Skills, something lasting begins to grow—the Life Skills they'll carry with them long after childhood.

Growing Skills are part of the learning stage, but Life Skills are the everyday habits, attitudes, and confidence that become second nature to your child. That's what makes Food Positivity more than an approach—it's the lasting Life Skill of relating to food and bodies with safety, trust, and joy.

Food Positivity looks like:

- Recognizing and responding to hunger and fullness cues
- Enjoying food without guilt, shame, or pressure
- Respecting that every BODY and every way of eating is valid and worthy
- Taking pride in their cultural foods while respecting those of others
- Questioning outside messages and filtering them through their own values
- Making decisions that align with their well-being, not outside pressure
- Connecting food to stories of science, culture, and community
- Seeing food as something to explore and discover, not just consume

And it doesn't end at the table. Food Positivity strengthens other core life skills like self-awareness, emotional regulation, critical thinking, problem-solving, and resilience. Research shows these skills are protective. They help kids navigate a noisy world with confidence, compassion, and respect for themselves and others.

Just like our kids, many of us are still practicing our own Growing Skills as parents—unlearning diet culture messages and building new ways of relating to food and bodies. That's not failure; that's growth. Every time you model resilience, curiosity, or compassion, you're showing your child that learning is lifelong, and that's one of the most powerful lessons you can give them.

Feeding Foundations: Food Positivity Life Skills

Food Positivity shows up across every part of your child's life, but it begins with eating. In the Feeding Foundations, it takes shape through daily routines and mealtime moments, where kids begin to turn practice into lasting confidence.

Food Positivity (Life Skill)

Eating with ease, trust, and joy.

Food Positivity is where all the Growing Needs and Growing Skills come together at the table. It's more than trying new foods—it's the lived experience of eating with ease, trust, and joy. Food feels safe. Bodies feel trustworthy. All foods and traditions have a place at the table. For kids, that means meals aren't about pressure, guilt, or rules— they're about connection, curiosity, and care. Their brain and body get the message: *Food is safe. My body is good. Eating is something I can enjoy.*

When eating feels stressful or uncertain—which all kids experience at times—Food Positivity offers us a way forward. Kids may feel judged for their food preferences, anxious with unfamiliar foods, or self-conscious about how much they eat. Without support, these moments can chip away at trust between you and your child, making mealtimes feel tense instead of building connection.

But when we nurture Food Positivity daily through the Growing Skills, everything shifts. Mealtimes become calmer, and kids show up with more openness and ease. Curiosity replaces fear. They stop when they're full, savor dessert without guilt, explore new foods with confidence, and take pride in meals that reflect their family and culture.

Everyday Moments That Support Food Positivity
- Making mealtimes a space for connection and fun
- Talking about food in neutral, curious ways instead of labeling it "good" or "bad"
- Noticing and honoring when your child says they're full—even if it's their favorite food (we'll get into the details of strategies like these in Part IV!)

Food Positivity Looks Different for Every Child

Food Positivity isn't about reaching one "perfect" way of eating; it's about supporting kids to engage with eating in a way that feels right for them. For some kids, especially those with Avoidant/ Restrictive Food Intake Disorder (ARFID), sensory sensitivities, autism, Attention-Deficit/Hyperactivity Disorder (ADHD), or a history of food trauma, Food Positivity might look very different. They might:

- Rely on a small list of safe foods
- Need more time and repeated exposures before trying something new—sometimes months or years
- Eat separately from the family at times to feel safe
- Struggle to notice hunger and fullness cues or respond to them consistently

This doesn't mean they aren't learning or growing. In fact, every experience of safety, trust, and choice at the table helps them feel more secure in their relationship with food—even if it doesn't lead to eating new foods right away. We'll work through specific strategies to help you support a child with feeding differences in Chapter 13.

Bringing It Home

You don't need to have all the answers or do everything "right" to raise a confident, curious eater. Just by showing up, noticing what your child needs, and approaching meals with care, you're already laying the foundation.

And it's okay if mealtimes feel messy or hard sometimes. Growth rarely follows a steady path. What matters most isn't whether your child eats the broccoli today but whether they feel safe and supported enough to stay open to trying it again when they're ready—knowing that taste buds can change.

You're not just feeding your child's body. You're shaping how they *feel* in that body. You're building trust. And every time you offer a meal without pressure, honor their "no," or let go of the clean plate rule, you're reinforcing that trust.

The work you're doing matters. And even when it feels small, it's adding up to something big.

Because that trust is in place, something powerful happens: Your child becomes more open to learning from you, the Food Leader.

One Simple Step

This week, try one small shift that builds connection over control. Maybe it's serving a "safe" food your child enjoys. Maybe it's letting your child explore something new with their hands. Maybe it's simply saying, "You don't have to eat it. You can just explore." You don't have to do it all. One moment of trust is enough to start.

Your Food Positivity Practice

Mealtime Moments: *Small Shifts to Pause & Grow*

6

The Building Blocks of Everyday Kids' Nutrition

All my son wants to eat is carbs! He'd live on cereal, rice, and naan if I let him. And he's always begging for sugar. I know it's not healthy for him to eat that way, so I've started buying low-carb wraps, cooking with cauliflower rice, and loading every meal with protein. But he's still obsessed, sometimes even sneaking cookies and crackers when I'm not looking. We're both cranky and tired, and lately he hasn't even been gaining weight. I'm just trying to serve him healthy food and help him understand there's more to life than carbs! What could I be doing wrong?

—Nisha

Now THAT WE'VE learned how to feed your kids in a way that builds trust and connection, you might be wondering: *But what about nutrition?* What do kids actually need to grow, thrive, and feel their best?

We get it, there's so much noise out there. One minute it's all about protein. The next, sugar is the villain. And somewhere in the middle, you're just trying to pack a lunch your kid will actually eat.

That's why this chapter is all about clearing the confusion and giving you real, practical information rooted in science *and* compassion. There's no such thing as "perfect" nutrition, but you can feel more confident making decisions that fit your child's needs, your family's core values, and your real life.

We'll walk you through the big picture of what helps kids feel full, energized, and satisfied. You'll learn how to think about balance, not just in terms of food groups but in terms of your child's appetite, activity level, and emotional needs, too.

Nourishing your family isn't about one meal or even a single day. It lives in the snacks you pack for the park, the last-minute freezer meals on busy nights, the comforting bowl of rice after a tough day, and the curiosity of a child exploring a new flavor for the first time.

A Balanced Diet Doesn't Mean What You Think

It's 5:45 p.m. You're staring into the fridge, three hungry kids behind you, each with totally different taste buds, and the only vegetable in sight is a lonely jar of pickles. Welcome to real life.

Diet culture would have us believe a balanced meal means a Pinterest-worthy rainbow of organic produce on every plate and not a processed item in sight.

But here's the truth: "Balance" doesn't live on a single plate. It lives in the rhythms of consistent meals and snacks and in the patterns of variety that you build over time. Even too much of one "good" thing (yes, even broccoli!) can crowd out other nutrients growing bodies need.

When you offer a range of foods across days and weeks, you're meeting your child's needs in a way that actually works for *real* life and for their *real* development. Supported by the reliable structure you'll provide as the Food Leader (more in Chapter 12), kids' bodies know how to use what you give them.

As parents, it's easy to worry that if you don't insist on two more bites of chicken, your child won't get enough protein. That fear makes sense with all the noise about what kids "should" be eating. But research shows that when parents offer consistent meals featuring a variety of foods, most children (without medical concerns) eat enough over time to grow and thrive. You don't need to micromanage bites; you need to lead.

So, what should you serve? That's entirely up to your family. What matters is that food is:

- Accessible and enjoyable
- Nutrient-rich and varied over time
- Aligned with your lifestyle and culture
- Offered in a way that respects your child's autonomy

As your family's Food Leader, the rhythms you create (predictable meals and snacks) and the patterns you build (offering a mix of foods without pressure) help your child feel safe, nourished, and able to tune into their own needs. They don't need "perfect" meals. They need steady variety, safe structure, and permission to listen to their bodies.

Balance is a rhythm of reliable meals and snacks repeating day after day and a pattern of varied foods that helps your child get enough of every nutrient across days and weeks.

It's not about getting it "right" every meal.

Remember, your cultural foodways belong here. Rice and beans. Injera and lentils. Dumplings and noodles. All of these have an important place on the plate. Nutrition and culture work together, not against each other.

Let's Talk About "Moderation"

When parents first hear about our work, they often say, "Yes! All foods fit—in moderation." We love the spirit behind that phrase (no food is off-limits), but you won't hear us use it.

On the surface, it sounds reasonable, even neutral. Yet "moderation" often keeps diet culture rules alive. It whispers that some foods are only okay in small amounts or that enjoying them too much makes you "bad." Same shame, softer packaging.

It's also incredibly vague. What counts as moderation? One cookie? Two? Once a day? Once a week? With no clear definition, it leaves parents second-guessing themselves and kids wondering if they've done something wrong. When we tack "in moderation" onto "all foods fit," we undercut the message. We're still hinting that certain foods are risky and need tight control.

Instead, we want kids to moderate their *own* intake. With time, consistency, and repeated exposure to eating patterns that support their growth (plus the occasional uncomfortable eating experience from too much Halloween candy, for example!), they will naturally learn to tell when enough is enough all on their own. They won't need the external control of "all things in moderation" because they'll be able to determine whether one cookie or two—or five!—is the right fit for them at any given moment.

When we move away from moderation as a rule and embrace structure and trust instead, we unlock true balance and give kids the tools they need for life.

Research Spotlight: The Surprising Path to Good Nutrition

It may come as a surprise given our "eat this, not that" culture, but decades of research show that strict food rules and restrictive diet plans usually *don't* result in high-quality diets. What does? A healthy relationship with food.

Studies from Ellyn Satter, Tracy Tylka, and other researchers have found that people who trust their hunger and fullness allow themselves to enjoy all kinds of foods and eat without guilt or pressure actually end up with higher quality diets and better health outcomes.

So instead of chasing food rules, chase joy, satisfaction, and balance—the nutrients will follow!

What Kids Really Need from Food

If you've ever fed a young child, you know their eating can feel like a roller coaster. One day it's endless pasta; the next, they seem to live on air. Bananas might be their favorite food, until the minute you buy a bunch, and then they sit browning on the counter. For parents used to tracking nutrients or chasing "five-a-day" checklists, this chaos can feel unnerving. How do you plan nourishing meals when your child's preferences change by the hour?

The answer isn't tighter control; it's zooming out. Instead of judging every bite or even every day, look for patterns over time. What matters most is that kids are *consistently* offered a variety of foods in a calm, pressure-free way.

That's where the three macronutrients come in: protein, fat, and carbohydrates. Sure, diet culture will tell you to focus on things like antioxidants or "brain-building" omega-3s, and those are important too. But macronutrients are the foundation of a well-rounded diet for both kids and adults. Knowing how each one supports growth, play, and focus and noticing how they naturally appear in everyday foods helps you build plates that nourish without moralizing food or adding stress.

We're not aiming for exact portions. We're after a flexible pattern anchored by structure, not rules. It's time to rethink "eating well" through a lens of evidence, body trust, and real-life flexibility.

So let's look at how protein, fat, and carbs work together for growth, energy, and satisfaction.

And as we'll emphasize in the remainder of this book, kids don't need nutrition facts; they need positive food experiences and trusted leadership from their grownups. The details that follow are for your confidence as the Food Leader, not your child's lesson plan. We'll cover how to talk to kids about food and nutrition in the next chapter.

Remember, you don't have to memorize every number or panic when the plate looks beige. Show up with consistency, curiosity, and care, and we'll take the rest one bite-size piece at a time.

Macronutrients: The Building Blocks of Everyday Nutrition

Macronutrients are the nutrients kids need in large amounts each day because they're the ones that provide energy (calories). When your child says they're hungry, it's usually macronutrients their body is asking for.

Carbohydrates, protein, and fat each play a different role in supporting your child's growth, focus, energy, mood, and movement. Together, they help fuel play, learning, and emotional regulation.

The good news is that you don't have to count grams or hit exact targets. Most foods contain a mix of macronutrients, and when you offer a variety of foods over time, you're likely covering what your child needs.

Bonus Handout via the QR Code: Nutrient Cheat Sheet

Protein: Building and Repairing Bodies

Protein helps kids grow, heal, build strong bodies, and stay satisfied after meals. It supports everything from immune function to tissue repair.

But here's what diet culture doesn't tell us: Most kids already get more than enough. Even if your child is going through a picky eating phase, isn't a big fan of meat, or has food preferences that limit variety, it's likely they're still meeting their protein needs. For example, a six-year-old's daily needs (just 19 grams!) could be covered by a glass of milk (8g) and a peanut butter sandwich (13g). It adds up quickly; no protein powders required.

> **Found in:** Animal sources such as beef, pork, chicken, turkey, fish, eggs, and dairy products. Plant-based sources include beans, lentils, tofu, edamame, nuts, and seeds.

Still, thanks to messaging that makes it sound like protein is the most important element of every meal, many parents worry their kids aren't getting enough. But protein doesn't have to be the main character at every meal or snack—it just needs to show up throughout the day. More protein isn't always better, especially if it replaces the carbs and fats that provide energy.

Daily Protein Needs

  1–3 years: ~13g/day (5–20% of daily calories)

  4–8 years: ~19g/day (10–30%)

  9–13 years: ~34g/day (10–30%)

In fact, if kids don't get enough energy from carbohydrates and fat, their bodies start using protein for fuel instead of what it's really meant for: growth and repair. This is called the protein-sparing effect, and it's one of many reasons balance matters.

Fat: Fuel for Growing Brains and Bodies

For years, fat has been misunderstood, avoided, and labeled "bad" by diet culture. But for kids it plays a vital role in supporting brain development, hormone production, immune function, and the absorption of key vitamins like A, D, E, and K. It's also the most calorie-dense macronutrient, which means it offers a lot of energy in a small package, especially important for kids with small stomachs and big needs.

And let's not forget: Fat makes food *taste* good! It helps kids feel satisfied and contributes to the flavor, texture, and enjoyment of meals—an often overlooked part of what helps kids stay nourished *and* build body trust.

Different Types of Fat (and Why Variety Matters)

There's no need to fear fat, but there's also no need to overcomplicate it. Fat isn't typically the "main" part of the meal; it's usually in other foods, like meat, eggs, or dairy, or added during cooking in the form of oils, butter, or spreads. This means you likely don't have to put much extra effort or planning to meet your child's fat needs.

Each type of fat plays a different role in your child's health, and their names describe the structure of fat molecules.

Monounsaturated Fats

Helpful for keeping cholesterol levels low and absorbing vitamins, these are often the easiest to incorporate into everyday meals.

Found in: Avocados, olive oil, canola oil, peanut butter, almonds, cashews, olives, hummus, dark chocolate

Polyunsaturated Fats

This group includes **omega-3** and **omega-6** fatty acids, essential fats that the body can't make on its own.

Omega-3s are especially important for brain and eye development, and they're often under-consumed in kids' diets, so it's important to offer foods with omega-3s regularly.

Found in: Salmon, tuna, sardines, flaxseed, chia seeds, walnuts, canola oil

Omega-6s   support skin, immunity, and overall growth.

Found in: Soybean oil, corn oil, sunflower oil, tofu, nuts, seeds, and many packaged foods

You might've heard omega-6s are "bad" or "pro-inflammatory," but current research shows that when eaten in balance with other fats, they're not harmful. This is just another way diet culture creates unfounded fears.

Saturated Fats

These fats are solid at room temperature and are recommended in smaller amounts (less than 10% of total calories), but most children will stay within a healthy range so long as they're offered a variety of foods that also include unsaturated fats.

Found in: Full-fat dairy (milk, cheese, yogurt), meat, eggs, butter, coconut milk, cream

Daily Fat Needs

1–3 years: 30–40% of daily calories

4–18 years: 25–35% of daily calories

Younger kids need more fat than older kids because of how rapidly their brains and bodies are developing. That's why breastmilk is naturally rich in fat and infant formula mimics this nutrient profile: It's nature's design.

As toddlers shift to table foods, they often continue getting enough fat through full-fat milk, yogurt, avocado, eggs, nut butters, and oils used in cooking. After age 4, many kids can safely transition to lower-fat dairy if their overall diet includes enough variety, but full-fat options can still be helpful and satisfying for many families.

Carbohydrates: The Unsung Hero of Childhood Nutrition

Fear-mongered and criticized, diet culture has long encouraged us to avoid carbohydrates, linking them to weight gain, sugar highs, or low-nutrient foods. But carbs are absolutely essential, especially for kids.

Carbohydrates are our body's preferred source of energy and the brain's primary fuel. Kids rely on carbs all day long—to run, climb, focus, regulate their emotions, and grow. When children don't get enough carbohydrates, they may feel tired, irritable, foggy, or struggle to concentrate. Limiting carbs in the name of "healthy" eating may actually mean withholding the very energy their growing bodies and brains rely on most.

When your child eats carbohydrates, their body digests them and turns them into glucose, a form of sugar that fuels everything from thinking and moving to healing and playing. That might sound surprising, especially if you've been taught to fear sugar. But glucose isn't a villain. It's the body's go-to energy source, and relying on it as the primary source of energy is exactly how the body is designed to work.

Different Types of Carbohydrates (and Why Variety Matters)

Not all carbohydrates act the same way in the body, and that's a good thing! There are a few different types, and each plays a unique role in helping kids feel energized, full, and regulated.

Simple Carbohydrates

Simple carbs are made up of one or two sugar molecules, which means the body breaks them down and digests them quickly. They provide energy right away, which is ideal for active kids or snack time when the next meal isn't far off.

Found in:
Naturally occurring sugars like those in fruit, milk, and yogurt
Added sugars like those in cookies, granola bars, flavored drinks, and some cereals

From a metabolic standpoint, our bodies break down all sugars into glucose, but natural sugars often come packaged with fiber, vitamins, and minerals, while added sugars do not. The issue with added sugars isn't that they're toxic. It's that when we consume them in large amounts, they can crowd out other important nutrients.

That said, we don't need to fear sugar. When we offer it regularly, without restriction or shame, our kids are more likely to learn to enjoy it in a way that makes their bodies feel good. This actually *decreases* the likelihood that they'll regularly consume so much sugar that it crowds out other nutrients.

EXPERT INSIGHT When Sugar Saves Lives: A Pediatric Dietitian's Perspective

Marina Chaparro, MPH, RDN, CDCES, of @nutrichicos and the Messy Bites podcast

As a pediatric registered dietitian living with type 1 diabetes—and counseling families who face it too—I've developed a very different perspective on sugar. For us, sugar can literally be life-saving during a low blood sugar episode.

In fact, a common medical recommendation is to treat hypoglycemia (low blood sugar) with 15 grams of fast-acting sugar in the form of glucose tablets, juice, or even candy. I once worked with a child who would intentionally try to go low, because that was the only time his parents allowed him to have sugar. That moment of joy was tied to an emergency, not everyday freedom. I've seen how this fear and constant restriction makes children crave it even more and how joy around sugar sometimes shows up only in extremes.

Complex Carbohydrates

Complex carbs are made of longer chains of sugar molecules, which means they take longer to digest. They provide steady energy and help kids stay full between meals.

Found in:
Starches: Bread, rice, pasta, potatoes, corn, peas, and beans
Fiber: Fruits, vegetables, whole grains, legumes

Yes, even starches like white bread, white rice, and regular pasta are *complex* carbohydrates! The way that grains are processed or refined can lead to digest them more quickly in some cases, as processing typically removes some of the fiber. But it's absolutely a myth that these foods are "basically sugar."

Fiber

Fiber is a special type of carbohydrate that the body can't fully break down. That might sound like a bad thing, but it's actually one of fiber's greatest strengths. Fiber helps support digestion, stabilizes blood sugar levels, and supports a healthy gut.

There are two kinds of fiber:
Soluble fiber, like oats, apples, and beans, slows digestion and helps lower cholesterol and keep blood sugar steady.
Insoluble fiber, like berries, whole wheat bread, and brown rice, adds bulk to stool and helps food move through the digestive system.

Most kids don't get enough fiber. A simple way to estimate your child's daily fiber needs is to aim for their age + 5 grams (for example, a 6-year-old needs about 11 g/day). You don't have to overhaul your pantry to add more fiber. Small additions like topping cereal with berries; adding salsa to eggs; choosing whole-grain snacks like popcorn, nuts, or seeds; or even serving fruit with the skin on can add up quickly.

What About Pairing Carbs with Other Nutrients?
Carbohydrates provide quick, ready-to-use energy. But when they're paired with protein, fat, or fiber, we digest them more slowly, which helps the energy they provide last longer and keeps kids feeling satisfied between meals. This is why a snack like crackers and cheese or toast with peanut butter works so well, because it's not just about filling our kids' bellies, it's about helping them stay energized and focused. So, if your kiddo seems to "crash" after a carb-heavy snack, consider adding a protein or fat source next time to help them stabilize their energy.

It might seem helpful to say some foods give us "quick" energy and others give "slow" energy, but for kids still learning to listen to their bodies, those labels can cause confusion and even create hidden food rules. We'll dive deeper into why in Chapter 9.

Daily Carbohydrate Needs

Carbs should make up 45–65% of a child's daily calories.

Children ages 1–18 need at least 130g of carbs per day, with most needing 200–250g or more depending on age, activity level, and growth.

Carbohydrates are not just "okay" to eat; they're actually *supposed* to make up a big portion of a child's diet!

Micronutrients: The Big Impact of Small Nutrients

We've talked about the major building blocks (carbs, protein, and fat), but there's a whole cast of behind-the-scenes helpers that keep your child's body running smoothly. These are the micronutrients, the vitamins and minerals kids need in small amounts to grow, learn, move, and thrive.

That doesn't mean you need to count every milligram or Google every food label. (*Please don't!*) Most kids (yes, even picky eaters) can get what they need when we offer a variety of familiar, nourishing foods consistently over time. That said, there are a few nutrients that deserve a little extra attention in childhood, either because they're more likely to fall short in kids' diets or because they play especially important roles during growth spurts and early development.

Iron   Iron helps carry oxygen in the blood and supports brain development, especially important during early childhood when the brain is growing fast. Low iron levels can lead to fatigue, trouble focusing, and a higher risk of anemia. Iron-rich foods include red meat, poultry, beans, lentils, iron-fortified cereals, tofu, and spinach. To maximize your child's iron absorption, pair iron-rich foods with a source of vitamin C like strawberries, citrus fruit, or bell peppers.

Calcium   Calcium builds strong bones and teeth, which is critical during childhood and adolescence when the body is building its lifelong bone bank. Calcium-rich foods include milk, yogurt, cheese, fortified plant milks, tofu, and leafy greens.

Vitamin D   Vitamin D helps the body absorb calcium and also plays a role in immune support. It's tricky to get enough from food alone, especially in areas with limited sun exposure. Vitamin D–rich foods include fortified milk, cereal, orange juice, eggs, salmon, and tuna. If your child doesn't get much sun, has a darker skin tone, or drinks plant-based milks, you might talk to your pediatrician about the need for a supplement.

Potassium   Potassium helps with muscle function, hydration, and keeping blood pressure steady. It's one of the nutrients most kids don't get enough of, mainly because many kids don't eat enough fruits and vegetables each day. Potassium-rich foods include bananas, potatoes, oranges, beans, yogurt, sweet potatoes, and tomatoes.

A Few More Nutrients Worth Knowing

These nutrients are commonly under-consumed by kids in the United States, especially those who eat a limited variety or struggle with food access.

- **Zinc:** Supports wound healing and immunity (meat, seeds, beans)
- **Choline:** Essential for brain development and memory (eggs, soy, chicken)
- **DHA:** An omega-3 fat for brain/eye development (salmon, fortified eggs, or milk)
- **Magnesium, Vitamin A, Folate, Vitamin K:** Often under-consumed but easily supported with small additions of beans, leafy greens, dairy, and whole grains

---

Processed Foods Are Not the Enemy

Let's talk about the P word: **processed**.

For many parents, "processed" has become code for "unhealthy," "lazy," or "bad parenting." But that's diet culture talking.

In reality, *most* foods are processed in some way. Bread, yogurt, applesauce, frozen veggies, canned beans, and even granola bars or chicken nuggets. . .they've all been processed to make them safe, convenient, or longer-lasting. And processing can actually make foods *more* nourishing, like when milk is fortified with vitamin D or cereal with iron.

So what do processed foods really do for us?

- Provide key nutrients (many are fortified)
- Make life easier for families with busy schedules
- Normalize real-world eating experiences for kids

Yes, some processed foods are higher in added sugar, fat, and sodium, and lower in the nutrients kids need to thrive. If these foods replace most of the nutrient-rich foods in a child's diet, that can affect a child's physical health. But even then, we have to remember that overall health is shaped by so much more, including social determinants like access, income, and support. Looking at the *Whole-Child*, raising healthy kids is about more than controlling what goes on their plates. It's about showing kids that all foods have a place and helping them learn to navigate them without shame.

Here's the takeaway: processed foods are not "poison," and they're not "devoid of nutrition." They provide energy, enjoyment, and convenience, and for families facing food insecurity, energy-dense processed foods can even be lifesaving.

That's why we push back on statements like, "We prioritize our kids' health, so we don't eat processed foods." The reality is every parent makes food decisions based on their circumstances and access. As we learned in Part I, for some, prioritizing their kids' health *is* putting processed foods on the table.

When we shame processed foods, we send the message that families who rely on them (including us!) are "less than." And when our kids enjoy them, this shame teaches them to distrust their own bodies instead of learning how to navigate all kinds of foods with curiosity, balance, and without guilt.

The goal isn't to avoid processed foods. It's to raise kids who can trust their bodies, enjoy food, and grow up confident making choices in a world where processed foods are part of everyday life.

__*Bonus Handout via the QR Code:*__ Real-Life Nutrition: Easy Wins for Busy Families

Bringing It Home

You don't have to be a nutrition expert to nourish your child well. When you understand the building blocks of nutrition and how different foods nourish the body, how balance supports well-being, and how satisfaction matters just as much as fiber or iron, you can approach meals with confidence, flexibility, and trust.

Nutrition isn't about perfect-looking plates or checking every box each day. It's about offering a wide range of foods over time, finding a rhythm that works for your real life, and remembering that feeding is about connection, not control. When you release the pressure to get it "right," you make room for curiosity, joy, and lifelong skills that matter more than any one meal.

One Simple Step

Notice one moment when you're tempted to control or "perfect" your child's eating. Take a breath. Say out loud: "Balance is a rhythm, not a rule."

Your Food Positivity Practice

Choosing New Food Language: *Letting Go of Old Scripts*

7

It Starts at Home: Your Most Powerful Tools for Raising Food and Body Confident Kids

My daughter has started refusing her snack before soccer practice. I finally found out that her friend said if you play on an empty stomach, you burn more energy and won't get fat. I insisted that she needs food for energy, but she pushed back and said it's not any different from how I usually skip breakfast. That is different though, because I'm trying to lose the baby weight from her two-year-old sister and she's actively growing. . .right? I'm not sure how to get her to see the difference.

—Lizette

FROM THE MOMENT they're born, kids are soaking up the world around them—watching, listening, exploring, and connecting. Every mealtime, grocery run, birthday party, and sideline snack becomes part of life's lessons. Whether we mean to or not, we're teaching them something about food and bodies every single day.

They're listening when we complain that our jeans feel tight. They're watching when we skip dessert or praise someone for "being good" because they ate a salad. They hear the coach joke about "earning" pizza with extra laps or see a TV ad calling a snack "guilt-free."

But they're also watching when we stop what we're doing to serve them a balanced meal and when we sit down to enjoy it with them. They notice when we casually mention that we just picked up a new pair of jeans because the old ones weren't comfortable anymore or that we say a fat joke on TV wasn't funny. These aren't just one-off moments, they're part of the environment that shapes how kids start to understand food, bodies, and themselves.

And the tricky part is, those messages aren't just coming from us. They show up everywhere, through grandparents, doctors, classmates, teachers, social media, food marketing, and even strangers in the checkout line.

Seeing the Bigger Picture: The Ecosystem of Food and Body Learning

"There are three teachers of children: adults, other children, and their physical environment."

—Loris Malaguzzi, founder Reggio Emilia approach
to early childhood education

All of these people, places, and experiences make up what we call the **Ecosystem of Food and Body Learning**. This web of influences shapes how kids see food, bodies, health, and identity.

The Ecosystem of Food and Body Learning

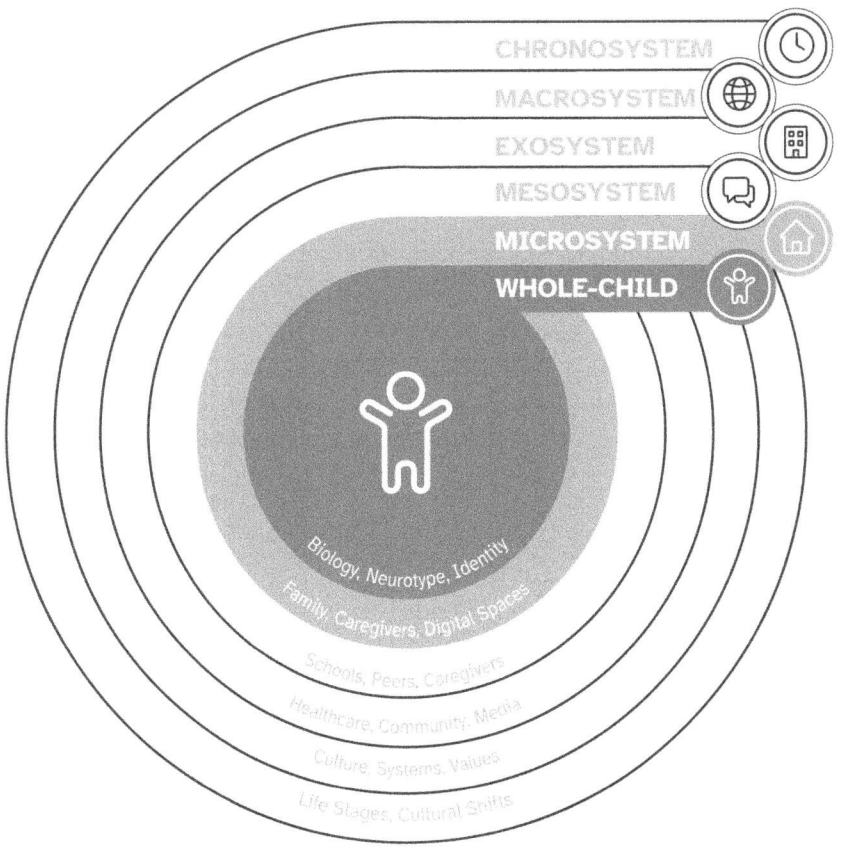

Research Spotlight: Where Food, Bodies, and Learning Intersect

This model is inspired by decades of research on how kids grow, learn, and form beliefs. It's based on Bronfenbrenner's Ecological Systems Theory and Bandura's Social Cognitive Theory. It also draws from neuroscience, trauma-informed care, and intersectional research that exposes the impacts of diet culture, anti-fat bias, racism, and ableism. We adapted these ideas for our modern world to focus on food and body learning so you can see the big picture of what's shaping your child's beliefs and where your voice matters most.

At the center of this ecosystem is your Whole-Child. They bring their own biology, sensory needs, identity, and lived experience to the way they learn.

Your child is always learning—at home, at school, and everywhere in between. And while you can't control everything they're exposed to, your voice is still the most powerful. The home environment is where kids learn how to interpret, question, and make sense of outside messages.

Your influence lives in everyday moments: how you talk about your own body, how you respond to dessert, how you comfort them when mealtimes feel hard. The conversations you have (and the ones you don't) shape your child's inner voice—how they feel in their body, what they believe about food, and whether they trust themselves.

You don't have to shield them from every message, because what you model at home becomes the filter they use to make sense of the outside ones. For example:

- When a teacher says, "Whole milk is unhealthy," a child from a food-positive home might wonder, "But why do we drink it at home?" and bring that question back to you, opening the door for curiosity and conversation.
- When a coach says, "We're running laps to burn off our pizza party," a child from a home where food is labeled or bodies are stigmatized might take it as proof that their body needs fixing.

That's why strengthening your child's at-home filter matters. This filter comes from your Family Core Values, the steady messages that guide how your child makes sense of the world. In Chapter 10, we'll talk about how to define and live out those values in daily life. In Part V, we'll look at how to support your child in navigating the wider ecosystem, like school settings and doctors' visits.

But right here, in the day-to-day of family life, what matters most is the environment you create at home. Even in a noisy world, a safe, supportive space and trusted adults can act as a child's compass. And that's exactly what the **Food Positivity Environment Foundations** are designed to provide.

The Food Positivity Environment Foundations

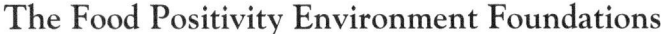

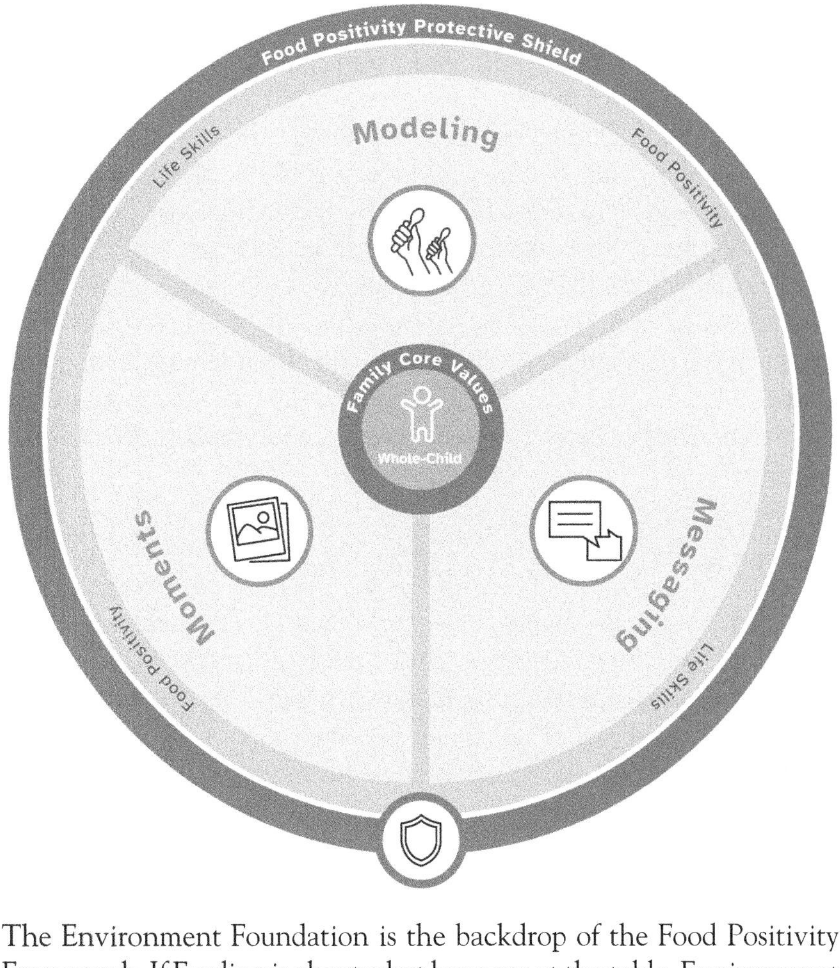

The Environment Foundation is the backdrop of the Food Positivity Framework. If Feeding is about what happens at the table, Environment is about what happens all around it. It's the setting that surrounds Feeding, Learning, and Parenting, shaping how your child experiences food and their body every day.

This is what we call the **Invisible Curriculum**—the everyday Modeling, Messaging, and Moments (3 Ms) that teach all the time, often without you realizing it. It shows up in the words you use about your body, the tone you bring to mealtimes, the routines that make food feel predictable, and the space you create for curiosity and care.

Because the environment never turns off, it weaves through every other foundation. It influences the needs your child feels and the skills they practice. When the environment feels safe and supportive, kids are more likely to explore new foods, trust their bodies, and build confidence that lasts.

Your child isn't just hearing your words; they're noticing your actions and how they feel in your presence. When those line up, the message is clear: "This is safe. This is how our family does things." But when they don't align, like saying "all foods fit" but also "I'm being good" when you decline dessert, it can leave kids feeling confused.

Once you start noticing the Invisible Curriculum, you'll see it everywhere: in mealtime rhythms, in the comments about bodies your child hears on TV, and in how you handle tricky moments at the table. And the best part is, once you notice it, you can start using it on purpose.

The 3 Ms—Modeling, Messaging, and Moments

The 3 Ms are always shaping your child's world. They affect how safe your child feels, how much they trust their body, and how adults meet their Growing Needs and support the development of their Growing Skills. Every look, word, and tone becomes part of the lessons they carry with them, not just at the table, but everywhere. We're going to start by looking at the 3 Ms through your child's eyes.

Modeling: What They See

Kids learn more from what we *do* than what we *say*.

If you make one dinner for yourself and another for your child because you're avoiding carbs, they notice. If you sigh at your reflection in the mirror, they notice. And when you all go out for ice cream with joy and without apology, they notice that too.

Modeling isn't about getting it right every time, especially if you're still working on your own relationship with food and your body (which is completely normal). It's about making choices with awareness. Every time you sit down and eat with your child, you're showing them that everyone deserves nourishment and enjoyment. Every time you choose not to criticize your body out loud, you're teaching them that bodies deserve respect.

Messaging: What They Hear

Words matter, especially for kids who are still figuring out just what they mean.

Because kids think literally, they often hear things differently than we intend. Even well-meaning comments can accidentally build fear or confusion (we'll learn why in Chapters 8!):

- "Sugar is bad." → They may believe *they* are bad for liking it.
- "Eat your veggies or you won't grow." → They may worry they'll actually stop growing.
- "No dessert until you finish dinner." → They may believe dessert needs to be earned.

And kids are listening even when we're not talking to them. Joking about being "bad" for eating chips, making comments about someone being too thin or too large, or even praising ourselves for eating a salad still sends a message.

You don't have to walk on eggshells. But once you notice the impact of your words, you can start using them to build trust, curiosity, and safety. (We'll dig into common "Food Talk Traps" and simple Food Positivity reframes in Chapter 9.)

Moments: What They Experience

This might be the most important M and also the easiest to miss.

Kids don't just remember what we fed them; they remember how they *felt* at the table. The pride of serving themselves, the joy of baking with you. The calm in your voice when their "no thank you" was enough. Those are the moments that stick.

And they also remember:

- Being called "too skinny" or hearing their body compared to others
- Being praised for finishing their plate
- The tension in your voice when they asked for seconds

These moments speak louder than any nutrition lesson or chart on the fridge. It's the tone, the feelings, and the emotional safety that leave the deepest mark. These are the lessons that last—and shape how they'll begin to think about food and their body for themselves.

When the 3 Ms line up and work together (what your child sees, hears, and feels), you harness the greatest influence they'll ever have: the environment you create at home. Yes, your child will have other influences. But what matters most is that home is the place where food feels safe, all bodies are good bodies, and they know they can always come to you. And that begins with you.

The Food Positivity Protective Shield

With the 3 Ms always at work, your child's Growing Needs supported, and their Growing Skills developing, your child begins to put Food Positivity into practice. And as they do, something even more powerful begins to grow: the Food Positivity Protective Shield.

This shield is your child's inner filter—the quiet, steady voice that helps them trust their body and question outside messages instead of accepting them as truth. It's the ability to pause and ask: *Does this fit with what I know about myself? Does this align with what I value?*

This shield grows layer by layer, moment by moment, through the safe, supportive, and respectful experiences you create at home—often in the small, ordinary moments that feel easy to overlook:

- Every time you honor their hunger or fullness cues. . .
- Every time you model body respect and speak kindly about food. . .
- Every time you affirm that their body and preferences are valued just as they are. . .

These moments—rooted in your values—add strength to the shield. Together they whisper to your child's brain and body: *I can trust myself. I am safe. I belong.*

And when the shield is strong, your child carries your voice and values with them wherever life takes them. They can:

- Hear a friend call a food "gross" and still enjoy it with pride
- Scroll past a fad diet and trust their hunger instead of chasing trends
- Hear someone say, "Eat a sandwich," and know their body is not up for debate

You can't control the Invisible Curriculum your child absorbs about food, bodies, health, or identity. But you can give them the filter they need to decide what to believe. That's how kids grow into adults who trust themselves, honor their needs, and make choices that support their well-being—no matter what the world throws their way.

Bringing It Home

Your home environment is always teaching through the words you say, the routines you create, and the way your child feels in your presence. The 3 Ms—Modeling, Messaging, and Moments—are the quiet teachers woven into daily life, shaping how your child learns to trust their body, explore food with curiosity, and carry Food Positivity forward.

Every time you pause to notice your words, align your actions, or create a calm, connected moment at the table, you're strengthening your child's Protective Shield. That shield becomes their inner filter, the steady voice that helps them trust themselves, question outside messages, and hold on to your family's values out into a noisy world.

Remember, this isn't about perfection. It's about showing up with intention, awareness, and care, one meal and one moment at a time.

One Simple Step

Choose just one "M" to notice today—Modeling, Messaging, or Moments. Watch how it shows up at meals, in casual conversations, or even during errands. What messages might your child be receiving, even if no one's "teaching"?

You don't have to fix anything, just begin noticing. Awareness is where transformation begins.

Your Food Positivity Practice

Building a Shield with the 3 Ms: *Everyday Choices That Protect Kids*

8

From Toddlers to Teens: What Kids Really Understand About Food and Bodies

The other day, my kindergartener ran straight into her room after school and turned off the lights. She took a book off of the shelf and squinted at it. "It's not working yet!" she said with disappointment. She later told me that she'd eaten all of her carrots at lunch and was hoping she'd be able to see in the dark by now. I just laughed, but it got me wondering where she heard that and what else she thinks food can magically do.

—Devon

FROM THE TODDLER who melts down over a PB&J sliced the "wrong" way to the preschooler who swears they don't like green foods to the tween who suddenly worries their body is "too big," you've seen how kids' understanding of food and bodies shifts as they grow. That means the way we support them has to shift, too, evolving right alongside them.

Kids are always learning, but not in the same way at every age. That's because kids aren't mini adults; they're meaning-makers. Their brains are still developing, and what might feel like a passing comment to you can be perceived as a hard truth or a rigid rule for them.

While every child is unique, there are predictable patterns in how children make sense of food, bodies, and social messages as their understanding deepens with age and experience. When we recognize these patterns, we can adjust what we expect kids to understand and how we teach them. Instead of oversimplifying, over-explaining, or assuming they "get it," we can respond with more compassion, more clarity, and a lot more calm.

Parent Reflection

Take a moment to pause. This chapter isn't about judgment or shame; it's about awareness. If you're feeling a twinge of guilt for how you've talked about food with your child in the past, remember: repair builds more trust than perfection ever could. You're learning while parenting. Your kids are learning as they grow. They don't need you to get it right every time; they just need you to keep showing up, with kindness toward them and yourself.

And chances are, you're already doing more of this than you realize. The goal isn't to overhaul your parenting but to notice what's working and build on it with intention.

In tough moments, try telling yourself: "Wherever I am today, it's not too late to change the tone of tomorrow." And if you're not sure how to start a new kind of conversation around food or bodies, start with something simple: "I learned something new today, and I want to share it with you."

That one line opens the door to connection, curiosity, and repair—exactly the conditions your child needs to feel safe enough to learn something new, too. At the end of this chapter, you'll find *Your Food Positivity Practice*, which will help you create your own version of that script and start shifting the conversation today.

Research Spotlight: Learning Through the Lens of Development

This chapter is grounded in decades of research on how kids grow, learn, and form beliefs about food and their bodies. We drew from developmental psychology, neuroscience, education, and nutrition science to better understand how children think at different ages, build trust and autonomy, and connect cause and effect.

Our approach blends best practices from Developmentally Appropriate Practice (NAEYC), Universal Design for Learning (UDL), and social-emotional learning, with insights from neurodiversity-affirming principles and sensory science. You'll also see ideas from classic developmental theorists like Piaget, Vygotsky, Bowlby, and Porges, as well as modern approaches like trauma-informed care and responsive feeding research. Again, we've distilled the science so you can focus on what matters most: supporting your child.

How Kids Make Sense of Food and Bodies

As you learned in Chapter 5, our kids' brains are still "under construction." They're constantly processing information and trying to make sense of what they hear, often filling in the blanks with the tools they currently have, like magical thinking, black-and-white logic, or ideas borrowed from others. That's why what we mean to teach isn't always what they actually learn. To us, their responses might sound silly, confusing, or even defiant. But really, it's just their developing brains at work.

Think about a preschooler covering their eyes while playing hide-and-seek and truly believing you can't see them because they can't see you. It's funny and sweet, and it's a perfect reminder of how kids are still learning to understand the world beyond their own perspective.

The same goes for food and bodies. Kids take in what we say (and what they hear elsewhere) and use their own developing logic to fill in the gaps. That's why the way they understand our words can look so unexpected and different from what we meant.

Let's take a look at a few of the most common real-life examples of how kids think and why those patterns matter when it comes to food and bodies.

How Kids Think (and Why It Matters)

Developmental Concept	How It Shows Up	Why It Matters
Egocentrism	Seeing the world from their own perspective and assuming others do, too.	If you diet or criticize your own body, they may assume something is wrong with *theirs* too, even if you never say anything directly about them.
Black-and-White Thinking	Understanding concepts in distinct extremes, like "good" or "bad," no in-between.	Labeling certain food as "healthy" may be understood as all other foods are "unhealthy" or "bad," which can lead to fear, guilt, or food rules.
Magical Thinking	Believing their wishes, thoughts, and actions can directly influence real-life.	A child might believe they got sick because they didn't eat their broccoli or that eating carrots gives them superhero eyesight instantly.
Concrete Thinking	Understanding the world in literal terms and focusing on what they can see, touch, or experience.	Kids need simple, real-world connections and cannot yet make sense of abstract ideas like "nutrients" or "balance."

Think of these concepts like a decoder ring: Once you know them, you can start to see what's really happening underneath your child's words and actions long before they have the language to explain it themselves.

But thoughts alone don't shape our kids' beliefs. As we learned with the 3 Ms, experience does. Every day, kids are learning from what they see, hear, and feel. And that's where your influence shows up most powerfully, in the tiny moments at the table, in the kitchen, or even at the grocery store.

Everyday Teaching Tools: How Beliefs Are Built

Teaching Tool	What It Looks Like	Why It Matters
Modeling	Kids copy what they see more than what they're told.	If you serve yourself veggies, talk kindly about your body, or try new foods, they're more likely to do the same.
Language (Messaging)	Words shape their beliefs.	Describing food as "junk" or "bad" can create shame, even if they enjoy it. What you say becomes their inner voice.
Repetition	Learning takes time and exposure, again and again.	Kids may need to see, smell, or hear about a food 15+ times before feeling safe enough to try it.
Sensory Experiences	Touching, smelling, and playing are part of learning.	Exploring food with all five senses, sparks curiosity, lowers fear, and builds familiarity, long before a bite happens.

(*continued*)

(*continued*)

Teaching Tool	What It Looks Like	Why It Matters
Playful Exploration	Imagination and creativity opens the door to discovery.	Pretending cauliflower florets are little sheep or making food faces turns pressure into play and play invites learning.
Routines	Predictability builds trust.	Regular meals and snack times teach kids that food is safe, needs are met, and nourishment is reliable.
Stories & Representation	What kids see in books, media, and conversations shapes their identity.	Books, media, and conversations that celebrate their culture, body, and food help kids feel like they belong.

It's Not "If" We Teach Nutrition, It's *How* and *When*

You might be wondering: "*But don't we still need to teach kids about food and nutrition? Wouldn't it be irresponsible not to? How else will they learn to make healthy choices?*"

The truth is you're already teaching them. As you saw in the previous chapter, kids are learning about food every single day through what you model, the words you use, and the everyday moments you create around eating—a.k.a. the Invisible Curriculum. Whether it's how you talk about your own body, the meals you bring to the table, or the tone you set at dinnertime, they're absorbing lessons all the time.

We're big believers in intentional food education, even for young kids (you'll see more on this in Chapters 9 and 20). But the key is keeping it developmentally appropriate. When you create learning opportunities that match how kids actually think, feel, and grow, you're building the foundation they need—the Needs and Skills that make space for curiosity now and allow for nuance later.

When we skip that foundation, our "nutrition lessons" don't land the way we intend. Instead of building understanding, they often turn into rigid food rules that do more harm than good. What you think is a simple fact about nutrients may be heard as: "If I don't eat this way, something is wrong with me or something bad will happen to me."

So instead of asking, "What can I teach my kids to make sure they eat healthy?" try asking, "How can I teach in a way that supports their development so they grow up knowing how to nourish themselves for life?"

Development 101: How Kids Understand Food and Bodies at Every Stage

If you've ever looked at your child and thought *What is even happening right now?* this section is for you.

Maybe they burst into tears because two foods were touching on their plate. Maybe they said, "I can't eat that; it's bad." Maybe they came home asking if eating fat makes people "fat." In the moment, those words and reactions can feel alarming. But most of the time, they're not signs that something is wrong, they're signs of growth. Each one is your child's way of testing big questions: *Am I safe? Do I belong? Can I trust my body and my grown-ups?*

Your child is learning, in real time, how to make sense of their body, their needs, and the world around them. When you understand what they're ready for at each stage—not just physically but emotionally and cognitively, too—you can shift from panic to care and from correction to connection.

This perspective helps you move beyond labels like "picky," "obsessed," or "disobedient" and instead see your child's behavior for what it often is: developmentally appropriate learning in progress. You stop expecting logic from a toddler or emotional regulation from a tween. You begin to see food refusal, rule-following, or body questions through a more compassionate lens.

That's why understanding *how* kids make sense of the world at each stage of development is one of your most valuable parenting tools. This section is your roadmap: When you use it to meet your child where they are, conversations feel smoother, power struggles ease, and you can guide their learning in ways that help shape what you want them to know about themselves and the world.

A Note on Development

These age ranges and stages are here to guide your understanding, not to serve as a checklist.

Kids grow and learn in their own ways. Some absorb lessons best through play or movement; others through repetition, stories, art, or hands-on exploration. Some pass through stages quickly, while others pause, regress, revisit, or take their own path.

This is especially true for neurodivergent kids, children with trauma histories, those in foster or adoptive care, or kids who've experienced food insecurity. They may need more time, more flexibility, and more Co-Regulation to feel safe around food and in their bodies. And that's not a flaw; it's just part of their story and their journey.

However your child learns, whatever stage they're in, the goal stays the same: help them feel safe, supported, and seen. That's why we ground this book in your child's foundational needs of Felt Safety, Co-Regulation, and Body Trust. When we focus *less* on control and *more* on connection, we make room for learning.

Early Childhood: 0–5 Years

Concrete thinkers. Sensory learners. Emotionally connected to their grown-ups.

Young children learn best through repetition, play, and connection. They don't need facts or lectures about food or bodies; they need safety, consistency, and trust. What they feel in their bodies and relationships now becomes the foundation for how they'll relate to food, hunger, and self-worth later.

Your role: Create calm routines, honor their "no," and let curiosity lead the way.

Infancy (0–12 Months)

The Big Learning at This Stage: Food is safety. My needs matter.

Every time you feed your baby, you're doing more than filling their belly; you're shaping what food and bodies feel like to them. Their brain is growing fast, fueled not just by calories but by rhythm, tone, and relationship. Even before starting solids, babies absorb the emotional experience of feeding: calm, connection, and trust. You're not just feeding them; you're teaching them: My *needs are worth honoring*.

How to Support Learning in Infancy

3 Ms	What This Looks Like	One Supportive Tip
Modeling	Your baby watches you eat and interact with food and your body.	Sit down to eat when you can. Let them see your face, your food, and your enjoyment.
Messaging	Tone matters more than words.	Use calm, rhythmic phrases like "You're hungry. Let's eat."
Moments	Feeding builds trust, safety, and co-regulation.	Allow mess and exploration, it builds sensory comfort and confidence.

Toddlers (1–3 Years)

The Big Learning at This Stage: Boundaries, big feelings, and the birth of autonomy.

Toddlers are discovering *I'm me, not you*. They explore that truth by throwing food, saying no, and changing their mind five times in a row. This isn't defiance; it's part of development. They're testing out what's safe, what's allowed, and how much control they really have over their bodies.

At this age, it's less about how many foods they eat and more about whether their "no" is respected. When we override their no, use food as a bribe, or respond with frustration, kids learn that eating is about performance, not trust. Your calm response is louder than any meltdown, it tells them, "You're safe, even when you say no."

How to Support Learning in Toddlers

3 Ms	What This Looks Like	One Supportive Tip
Modeling	Toddlers copy what they see, especially how you react.	Narrate curiosity: "Hmm, this smells sweet! It reminds me of grandma's plum pie" (no pressure to taste).
Messaging	Language shapes safety; keep it simple and validating.	Say: "You don't have to eat it" or "It's okay to be unsure."
Moments	Messy meals and food refusals are trust-building opportunities.	Stick with a calm, predictable routine. Toddlers thrive on structure.

Preschoolers (3–5 Years)

The Big Learning at This Stage: Imagination, identity, and all-or-nothing thinking.

Preschoolers are full of big questions, but they're still concrete thinkers. Their brains crave order, so they naturally sort the world into simple categories: letters versus numbers, girls versus boys, good versus bad, healthy versus unhealthy. They often repeat what they hear, even without fully understanding it because they're testing how those ideas fit with what they already know.

This is also when their identity stories start to form: "I'm a good eater." "I'm a picky eater." "I never finish my dinner."

These little stories stick. They shape how kids see themselves in relation to food and their bodies. As peers begin to influence their thinking, your voice still carries the most weight, especially when you respond with curiosity and care. By helping your child question the messages they hear, you're helping them shape the ability to think for themselves.

How to Support Learning in Preschoolers

3 Ms	What This Looks Like	One Supportive Tip
Modeling	They're watching how you talk about food, bodies, and yourself.	Show body respect out loud. Stretch, eat a variety of foods, and speak kindly about yourself.
Messaging	They take your words literally; sarcasm and moral labels are understood as truths.	Try: "That's crunchy! What does it taste like?"
Moments	They repeat what they hear; these are teachable, not shameable.	Ask: "What made you think that?" Then gently reframe the thought with compassion.

Understanding "Health" Is Still Too Big

At this age, kids don't actually grasp what the word *health* means; to them it's "what grown-ups say is good." That's because health is an abstract, future-oriented idea, and young kids don't think that way yet. Developmentally, they live in the here and now. So when

(continued)

(*continued*)

they repeat "This food is healthy," they're usually parroting back what they've heard, not making sense of it in their own way.

Instead of saying: "This is healthy."

Try: "This fills our bellies," or "This gives us energy to play."

Concrete, sensory-based phrases like these give kids information they can actually use right now, what they feel in their body, what they notice, what's true in the moment. That way, you're teaching without fear, morality, or pressure.

Middle Childhood: 6–9 Years

Concrete thinkers in a more complex world. Hungry for praise, fairness, and belonging.

Kids in this stage start noticing how others talk about food and bodies, whether at school, with friends, or on screens. They still see things in black-and-white, so words like *healthy* or *bad* carry a lot of meaning. But their memory and emotions are getting stronger, which makes this a golden window to build trust, affirm body respect, and guide their curiosity.

Your role: Help them make sense of what they see and hear by listening, asking questions, and gently reframing what they share.

Early Elementary (5–7 Years)

The Big Learning at This Stage: Rules, reasoning, and social signals.

Kids in this stage are learning how the world works. They want it to make sense. They're still concrete thinkers, but they're starting to understand cause and effect, fairness, and logic. And this is the age where they begin looking to peers for social cues and really start noticing how others talk about, label, and judge bodies.

They're also starting to understand emotions, and they care deeply about what trusted adults think and say. That makes your language especially powerful. So, if they hear things like "Sugar is poison" or "If you don't eat your veggies, you won't grow," they may take these messages as hard rules. This is the age when food rules start to solidify, but it's also the perfect time to reframe them before they become too rigid.

How to Support Learning in Early Elementary

3 Ms	What This Looks Like	One Supportive Tip
Modeling	They notice how you justify or judge food and body choices.	Normalize variety. Say: "Our bodies need all different kinds of foods."
Messaging	They want clarity and fairness; your words shape their beliefs.	Say: "Foods gives us energy," instead of labeling energy as quick or slow.
Moments	They may echo what peers or media say, so this is your chance to guide them.	Ask: "Where did you hear that?" Then gently explore the idea together.

Late Elementary (8–10 Years)

The Big Learning at This Stage: Comparison, logic, and testing what fits.

At this stage, kids are becoming more socially aware. They start comparing how they look, what they eat, and how they measure up to peers. They may repeat things they've heard from friends, media, or school about dieting, food rules, or body size, even if they don't fully understand what those messages mean.

Their cognitive development *is* expanding: They're asking more questions, making more connections, and starting to apply logic to what they've learned. But their emotional maturity hasn't caught up yet, which means your tone and context still matter.

This age is an important window where you can reinforce body diversity, Food Positivity, and trust in their inner cues before outside pressures grow much louder. Your steady, curious response shows them they don't need to be "right." They just need to be safe asking questions. When they repeat something that sounds concerning, it's an opportunity to start a new kind of conversation.

How to Support Learning in Late Elementary

3 Ms	What This Looks Like	One Supportive Tip
Modeling	They're watching how you speak about your body, others' bodies, and what "healthy" looks like.	Show gratitude for your body: "I'm thankful my legs let me play soccer with you."
Messaging	They repeat social messages they don't fully understand, especially around food and weight.	Ask: "Where did you hear that?" Then offer a calm, curious reframe.
Moments	Everyday comments shape identity and belonging.	Be their safe space. Normalize questions, even if they're uncomfortable.

Later Childhood to Adolescence: 10+ Years

Abstract thinkers forming their identities. Tuned in, even when they tune you out.

Tweens and teens are more independent, critical, and socially aware. They compare themselves to peers, question what they've learned, and interpret messages through a deeply personal lens. This is when food and body stories either solidify or start to unravel.

What they need most isn't control; it's connection. They need you to be their safe, nonjudgmental space where they can test out ideas, push back, and still know they're accepted. Even if they roll their eyes, your consistency guides them.

Your role: Stay close, stay curious, and let connection lead.

Tweens (10–12 Years)

The Big Learning at This Stage: Identity, independence, and internalization.

Tweens are shifting from black-and-white thinking into a more nuanced view of the world. They're beginning to internalize the messages they've absorbed about health, weight, food, and their bodies and ask: *What does this mean about me?*

They're forming their own opinions, but social pressure is rising. You might notice them experimenting with food rules or repeating things they've heard from peers, teachers, or media. And while they crave independence, they still need your steady presence to help sort through the noise.

This is a pivotal stage. The stories tweens build now become internal narratives they'll carry into adolescence and beyond. They still care deeply about what trusted grown-ups think, so when you validate their curiosity and hold space for the tough stuff, you remain their trusted guide even when the outside world gets louder.

How to Support Learning in Tweens

3 Ms	What This Looks Like	One Supportive Tip
Modeling	They're starting to question adult behaviors, even if they don't say it out loud.	Help them work through contradictions they notice, "What do you think about what you saw/heard?"
Messaging	They're testing what they've heard from peers, media, or school.	Say: "That's an interesting idea, where did you hear that?" Then learn about it together.
Moments	New experiences (think team snacks, locker rooms, cafeterias, and social media) spark big questions.	If they repeat something concerning, pause and ask: "What made you think that?"

Teens (13+ Years)

The Big Learning at This Stage: Critical thinking, comparison, and control.

Teenagers are deep in developing their identities. They're starting to think critically about the world and themselves. They want independence and privacy, but what they've absorbed earlier in life now shows up in more complex ways: food rules, body dissatisfaction, disordered eating patterns, or internalized beliefs about "health" and worth.

This is also when the world's messages about diet culture, weight stigma, and body ideals hit the hardest. Social media, school health classes, comparisons with their peers, and adult commentary all play a role, especially when teens feel pressure to perform or fit in.

But research shows that strong, trusting relationships with caring adults still matter most. Even if they act like they're not listening, even when you feel invisible, your presence helps them feel safe enough to question harmful messages and reconnect with their own body wisdom. The goal isn't to control your teen's choices. It's to stay connected enough that they'll turn to you when something doesn't feel right.

How to Support Learning in Teens

3 Ms	What This Looks Like	One Supportive Tip
Modeling	They're comparing your actions to your values and looking for authenticity.	Be honest about your growth: "I used to think that too. I'm still working on unlearning it."
Messaging	They're quick to detect judgment and may shut down if they sense it.	Reflect back their insight: "You've probably heard that a lot, what do you think about it?"
Moments	Real learning happens in small everyday moments like meals, car rides, and dog walks.	Stay close, not controlling. They'll open up when they feel emotionally safe.

<u>**Bonus Handout via the QR Code:**</u> At a Glance: How Kids Learn About Food and Bodies at Every Age

So What Does Teaching Kids About Food and Nutrition Look Like in Practice?

For toddlers, food and nutrition learning doesn't come from facts or charts; it comes from play. Dipping a hand into yogurt and yelling, *"It's cold and slippery!"* is just as important as tasting it. Making up a song about green beans around the table is how curiosity and confidence grow.

For preschoolers, it's still about stories and sensory play. They may not understand *why* carrots are orange, but they can describe them as "crunchy" or "sweet." These playful, concrete moments are the building blocks for trust and confidence around food.

By early elementary school, kids start noticing patterns and cause-and-effect. They might realize, "Rice fills my belly differently than a granola bar," or that salty snacks make them thirsty. These little observations are the beginnings of nutrition learning grounded in what their body feels, rather than memorized rules.

By the tween years, kids are ready to connect those lived experiences to more abstract ideas. A middle schooler who's learned about digestion and macronutrients might say, "I need both carbs and protein before soccer so I don't run out of energy." The difference is that they're not following a rule someone gave them in a classroom; they're making meaning from their own experience. That's when abstract nutrition concepts finally click, because the foundation has been laid.

When we let food and nutrition education grow alongside kids' development, it doesn't just teach them *what* to eat. It gives them Food Positivity Life Skills: trusting hunger and fullness cues, planning and preparing meals, making choices that feel good in their bodies, and approaching food with confidence instead of fear.

Bringing It Home

Understanding how kids think at each stage doesn't just help you parent; it helps you see your child with more compassion. It gives you tools to respond to what's *underneath* the behavior, not the behavior itself. It helps you meet your child where they are.

And this isn't only about your child's growth; it's about yours, too. As you read about how kids process food and body messages, you may have recognized echoes of your own story: the food rules you absorbed, the shame you carried, or the lessons you're still unlearning. That reflection matters. Raising food and body-confident kids often means offering yourself the same healing you want for them.

This is also where the Food Positivity Environment Foundations from Chapter 7 connect. Development shapes *how* your child understands messages; your home environment shapes *what* they do with them. Together, they form the Protective Shield your child needs to filter out the noise of diet culture and stay grounded in your Family Core Values.

You don't need to get it exactly right, and it's impossible to block out every outside message. What matters is that you keep showing up with curiosity, connection, and care. Each small moment strengthens that shield and gives your child the tools to pause, question, and choose the outside messages they believe instead of absorbing every message as truth.

One Simple Step

Connect to your child's age and stage. The next time your child does or says something around food or bodies that catches you off guard like refusing a familiar food, repeating a "diet-y" phrase, or asking a tough question, pause and ask yourself: *What might this mean for their age and stage?* That small pause to consider the *why* instead of reacting to *what* builds empathy, reduces conflict, and helps you respond in a way that truly supports their growth.

Your Food Positivity Practice
Starting Fresh: *A Simple Script to Build Connection*

9

Food Talk Traps: When Food Talk Teaches More Than We Mean

When my son was five, he always wanted to know how things worked. So when it came to food, we explained it factually. One thing we talked about was long energy and short energy foods and how protein helped make food have longer energy. But a few months into kindergarten, mornings became stressful. He would check his backpack again and again to make sure he had everything and panic about protein. He'd walk to the bus stop in tears, saying "Do you think I had enough protein? What if I'm hungry before lunch?" It became clear that he was struggling with anxiety and this gave him something to focus on. It was one more thing that he might be doing "wrong."

—Rebecca

NEARLY EVERY PARENT we know, including ourselves, has reached for some version of a "magic phrase" to convince a child to eat. We want our kids to eat nourishing foods instead of just desserts and snacks, so we reach for words that sound reasonable. . .until we realize they don't always land the way we hoped.

By now you know kids are always learning about food and bodies—that what you say matters, but what your child *hears* isn't always what you meant. And it's not because you've failed. It's because most of the scripts we were handed weren't designed with children's development in mind.

These lessons were passed down through decades of nutrition messaging, public health campaigns, school programs, and even social media "tips," all trying to make nutrition for kids feel simple. From the Food Pyramid to MyPlate to traffic-light charts and "quick versus slow energy," adults have leaned on easy categories that feel helpful to us. But kids don't process them the same way and what we're teaching them isn't always scientifically accurate.

Most of us grew up believing that eating well meant someone else knew better than we did—a parent, a diet plan, or a health expert. If you've never trusted your own body to self-regulate, of course you feel like you have to teach, convince, or control your child. But this is your opportunity to give your kids something different.

Let's pull back the curtain on those everyday "helpful" phrases that can unintentionally undermine your child's trust in their body.

Parent Reflection

As you read through these common Food Talk Traps, some may sound familiar. Maybe you've said them yourself. This isn't about blame. It's about noticing.

- What did I really mean when I used those words?
- What was I hoping my child would learn or do?
- What might my child have actually heard at their age or stage?
- Does that match what I really want them to understand?

The truth is good intentions can still teach unhelpful lessons. Most traps share the same root: trying to control or convince. The "old way" (pressure, fear, control) may bring short-term compliance, but it often leads to long-term resistance.

Kids aren't just eating; they're learning. And the way we talk shapes not only what they put on their plate but what they believe about food, their bodies, and themselves.

"Children naturally explore, learn, and grow. Warnings about food impede their exploration. To cope, they become rigid and try to live by rules that are to them illogical, ignore them completely, or give up and become rebellious."

—Ellyn Satter, *Secrets of Feeding a Healthy Family*

Food Talk Traps: When "Helpful" Words Become Harmful

Kids are natural meaning-makers. They don't just hear your words; they interpret them, store them, and build beliefs out of them. Over time, it adds up into a *pattern*, part of the Invisible Curriculum shaping how your child understands food and bodies.

The problem is many of these lessons are developmentally mismatched. What sounds fun or simple to us ("Green foods help you fight off sickness") can feel like a hard rule, a warning, or even a judgment to a child.

Think of it this way: Handing a preschooler a chapter book while they're still learning their ABCs doesn't help them learn to read faster. No matter how colorful the cover, they're simply not ready to make sense of it yet. The same is true for food talk. If the message doesn't match their stage of development, it can do more harm than good.

We hope to teach them to eat "better," but often end up setting them up for the same trap we fell into ourselves: believing that eating well means trusting someone else more than themselves.

EXPERT INSIGHT: When "Healthy" Messages Harm: A Pediatric Dietitian's Perspective

Elizabeth P. Davenport, MPH, RDN of @sunnysideupnutritionists & Pinney Davenport Nutrition

Diet culture is everywhere. We are bombarded with fear-based messages about food from all directions and taught to see them as "healthy."

(*continued*)

(*continued*)

Parents repeat this language because they've been led to believe talking about food this way will help their children be "healthy," too. But when the very messages we're passing on to our kids are grounded in food fears and worries about weight gain, that's confusing and often harmful to our kids.

A supportive first step is to start noticing the thoughts about food and nutrition that go through your mind and then practice *not* saying them aloud. If your children are older, you might let them know you're working on changing the way you talk about food and nutrition, because you learned that what you've been saying can be confusing to kids and teens.

And most importantly, parents can also remind themselves that they're not alone. Making changes in the way you talk about food and nutrition is a powerful way to support your children in having a positive relationship with food.

Trap 1: Binary and Dichotomous Thinking

"Healthy versus unhealthy." "Good versus bad." "Every day versus sometimes." "Go—slow—whoa." "Quick versus slow energy." "Real food."

Parents use these categories because they feel like simple guidance, and they're everywhere. But the tricky part is, young kids don't think the way adults do. They're literal thinkers. To them, a rule is a rule. Green means safe. Red means danger. A cookie in the red zone doesn't register as "sometimes"; it feels like a warning.

Because kids are also learning colors, symbols, and stop/go rules, visuals like traffic lights pack an even stronger punch. Instead of noticing when they're hungry, full, or curious, they start judging food by external rules (just like adults learned to do on diets). And when a food they love—or even a family staple—gets labeled "bad," the shame can extend beyond the plate, influencing how they feel about their body, their home, and their culture.

What starts out looking playful can quietly plant rigid ideas: Some foods make you "good," others make you "bad." Over time, that mindset becomes a gateway into restriction, fear, and shame.

Food Positivity Reframe: Kids don't need stoplights, moralizing scorecards, or hierarchies. They need language that builds trust and nurtures curiosity.

What You Said	What You Meant	What They Heard	The Hidden Takeaway	Food Positivity Reframe
"Healthy versus unhealthy."/ "Slow energy versus fast energy."	I want you to know some foods help your body feel good more often than others.	Red = danger. Green = safe. Some foods (and people who eat them) are good, others are bad.	Food is about rules and "goodness," not listening to my body. I should judge foods as better or worse instead of trusting myself.	"Different foods do different things for your body. All foods have a role. Eating eggs for breakfast keeps my tummy full until lunchtime. How about you?"

Why We Don't Teach "Quick" vs. "Slow" Energy

It might seem helpful to say some foods give "quick energy" and others give "slow energy." On the surface, it feels like a simple, "science-y" way to explain how food turns into fuel. But here's the problem: It's not accurate *or* developmentally helpful.

(continued)

(*continued*)

- **It's not reliable:** The idea comes from the glycemic index (GI), which ranks foods by how quickly they raise blood sugar. But in real life, food doesn't behave in simple categories. A banana's effect changes depending on how ripe it is. Pasta digests differently if it's firm (al dente) or soft. Add butter, and that slows things down again. And each child's body responds uniquely. Even more surprising is that chocolate cake is technically "slow energy" because fat and protein slow digestion, while watermelon counts as "quick energy" because its high water content makes sugar absorb faster. Those aren't exactly the lessons most parents are trying to teach their kids.
- **It overrides Body Trust:** When we tell kids how food *should* act, they stop noticing how it actually feels. Instead of asking themselves, "Did that snack help me keep running and playing?" or "Am I starting to feel hungry again?" they start relying on external influences on how foods *should* feel instead of tuning in.
- **It creates hidden food rules:** In practice, parents rarely call dessert "slow energy." That label gets reserved for the foods we *want* our kids to choose more often. That means "slow" quietly becomes code for "better," setting up another hierarchy that can leave kids feeling restricted or guilty.

The best nutrition lesson isn't about quick versus slow categories; it's about helping kids notice how food actually feels in their bodies so they can begin to build Food Positivity Life Skills.

Trap 2: Restriction, Scarcity, and Food Elevation

"That's junk." "These are sometimes foods." "You can't have dessert until you finish dinner." "This is a special treat." "Fun foods."

We often use restriction as a tool to encourage kids to eat more of the variety they need. These phrases may feel harmless and maybe even protective. It feels logical: If I teach my child why we limit sweets, they'll eat more of the "healthy" stuff.

But when we ration, restrict, or use food as rewards, they become more powerful in a child's mind. Dessert becomes a prize and vegetables become the "work" you have to get through to earn it. Labels like "junk" are even worse, equating foods they enjoy or foods a family can access, with trash. Calling something "special" or "fun" only elevates a food more, making them feel rare and extra desirable, while other foods feel boring or second-best by comparison.

And words like "sometimes" may sound flexible to us, but kids can't really process what that means. To them, it feels like rationing: *How do I know when it's okay? What if I mess up?*

Instead of reducing their interest in sweets or their sugar "obsession," restriction often feeds it. Kids sneak food, overeat in secret, or feel guilty for wanting what's "bad." Over time, they tune out hunger and fullness cues, and eating becomes about following rules (or rebelling against them).

When foods are sorted into forbidden, special, or better-than, kids don't learn balance. They learn mistrust of food, of their bodies, and sometimes. . .of us.

Food Positivity Reframe: When all foods have a place, kids feel calmer, more confident, and less "obsessed."

What You Said	What You Meant	What They Heard	The Hidden Takeaway	Food Positivity Reframe
"Finish your dinner to get dessert."/ "That's junk food."	I want you to get the nutrients you need before filling up on sweets.	Dessert is the best part. I have to earn it. My favorite foods are bad or wrong.	Some foods are more valuable than others. I need to sneak, overeat, or feel guilty about foods I love.	"All foods can fit on our plates. Tonight we'll have chicken, rice, peppers, and cookies."

Trap 3: Fear-Based and Shame-Inducing Narratives

"Sugar makes you hyper." "Sugar will rot your teeth." "Too much will make you fat." "You're going to get diabetes if you keep eating dessert that way."

Fear-based messages may also feel protective, like a warning to keep kids safe. But fear doesn't teach or build understanding; it creates anxiety. It may change what a child eats in the moment, but the lesson that lingers is shame and body distrust.

A child may eat sugar and notice no difference in how they feel. Then they learn that a friend with diabetes actually *needs* sugar when their blood sugar drops. They may hear that "sugar rots your teeth," but then watch adults enjoy dessert without consequence. When these lessons don't add up, kids get confused and that confusion can chip away at their trust in us and in themselves.

Threats tied to weight or illness send an even harsher message: *My body is risky, and I can't trust it.* For kids in larger bodies, smaller bodies, or those who already feel different, that message is even more harmful: *My body is wrong.*

The truth is most of these claims oversimplify or twist science. "Sugar highs" at parties? Research validates that it's the excitement of the celebration, not the sugar itself. Cavities? It's more about good dental hygiene, fluoride, and genetics than the cookie itself. And while food plays a role in health, chronic diseases come from many factors outside a child's control (think the SDoH!), and kids are not in control of their personal well-being anyway; that's the responsibility of the grown-up. Teaching otherwise isn't honesty; it's diet culture.

Food Positivity Reframe: Fear doesn't teach; it intimidates. Kids need honesty they can understand, delivered without shame.

What You Said	What You Meant	What They Heard	The Hidden Takeaway	Food Positivity Reframe
"Sugar will rot your teeth."/ "Too much junk will make you fat."/ "That food will make you sick."	I want you to be healthy and avoid health problems.	Sugar is dangerous. Fatness is bad. My body can't be trusted.	Eating is risky. My body is a problem to control. Food causes shame, not joy.	"Food gives your body energy and helps you grow. Let's notice how this food feels in your body."

"But I Just Want to Be Honest with My Kids. . ."

One of the most common concerns we hear is: "I don't want to sugarcoat things. I just want to be honest about food."

And you can be honest. But our honesty has to match what kids are ready to understand. Think about how we approach body safety: We use real, anatomically correct words for genitals because it protects kids and reduces shame. But we don't teach everything at once. We layer the information gently, in concrete ways kids can emotionally and cognitively handle.

Developmentally honest teaching sounds more like:

- "This snack is my favorite snack in the summer when my body feels sweaty and hot. What about you?"
- "This food gives us energy to run and play."
- "Our bodies need lots of variety. That's why I like having a mix of different foods throughout the day."

Trap 4: Oversimplification and Function Overpromising

"Carrots help you see in the dark." "Milk makes strong bones." "This is brain food." "Red foods are good for your heart." "Some do a little, some do a lot."

We say these phrases hoping if kids know the "why," they'll choose the "healthier" foods we want them to eat. But here's the problem: Young kids are just starting to learn body awareness and naming body parts; they can't understand body functions yet. Teaching food by function is like asking a five-year-old to solve algebra before they can count.

Because kids are magical, literal thinkers, they take these messages at face value. A preschooler with glasses might believe carrots will fix their eyesight. A child with asthma or leukemia may think they caused it because they didn't eat their vegetables.

And for kids who can't eat the "healthy" food being praised, the message can be especially harmful. A child with lactose intolerance who hears "Milk makes you strong" may believe their body is weak. A child with celiac disease who hears "Whole grains give you a smart brain" may think their brain will never be good enough or they'll never be as smart.

And if you have ever started down the road of "food function" talk with your kiddos, then you know kids often want to know what *every* food does. But in reality, foods don't have one simple job. Real food is complex. A banana isn't just potassium. A cookie isn't just sugar.

When we give foods "jobs," it sets up hierarchies where some foods "do more" meaning are good and have more moral value, while others are less valuable. "Food function" talk is simply diet culture's food policing, rebranded for kids. And the problem is, kids can start to feel like their safe foods, cultural or religious dishes, or even the foods that are easiest for their family to access aren't good enough.

When we reduce food to "jobs," eating becomes something kids "perform" to get praise, to be "good," or to accomplish a goal (grow tall, get strong, heal faster). Kids feel pressure to make the "right" choice instead of discovering what they enjoy most, how a food makes them feel, or actually connect it to how their body works.

Food Positivity Reframe: Food serves many roles: connection, comfort, culture, energy, growth, and joy. Function is just one part of the story.

The Problem with "Red Foods Are Good for Your Heart"

Parents nod along, thinking it's nutrition made easy. But it's not accurate *or* developmentally aligned.

- **Not all foods of the same color do the same thing:** "Yellow foods heal cuts" comes from vitamin C, but not every yellow fruit or veggie has vitamin C. Same with "Red foods are good for your heart." That idea comes from lycopene, a nutrient in tomatoes and watermelon. But other red foods, like strawberries or red cabbage, get their color from different nutrients that support health in their own ways. Grouping them together oversimplifies the truth and gives kids the wrong idea.
- **Oversimplification confuses kids:** Kids are concrete, literal thinkers. When they hear "Red foods are good for your heart," they may assume red lollipops or sports drinks count too. And if we get specific with fruits and vegetables, then we risk creating another hierarchy because we aren't talking about other foods the same way.
- **The message misses the point:** These playful phrases are really adult nutrition facts repackaged for kids. Oversimplifying doesn't make them developmentally appropriate; it makes them confusing, misleading, and sometimes flat-out wrong.

And yes, red fruits and veggies are nourishing. But if we want to build trust with our kids, honesty and accuracy matter just as much as the lesson itself.

What You Said	What You Meant	What They Heard	The Hidden Takeaway	Food Positivity Reframe
"Carrots help you see in the dark."/ "Food is fuel."	I want you to eat foods that help your body grow strong.	If I don't eat the "right" foods, my body won't work. Some foods are magical, others are useless.	I should eat to make my parents happy or prove my health. If I don't like certain foods, I'm failing my body.	"Food has many roles. It gives energy, helps your body grow, and can also be tasty, comforting, or part of a family tradition."

Trap 5: Exclusion and Erasure of Culture/Body Diversity

"Eat the rainbow." "Clean eating." "Real food." "Whole food." "Ingredient household."

At first glance, these messages sound positive. We use them because we want eating "healthy" to feel simple and fun. But when we look closer they often reinforce one narrow picture of health that leaves out entire cultures, classes, and bodies.

Take the phrase "Eat the rainbow," for example. It can be a helpful way to encourage variety, but it's usually taught with only fruits and vegetables, often leaving out many beige or brown staples like rice, potatoes, yucca, plantains, or taro. And even when all food groups are included, lessons regularly skip over everyday cultural dishes like curries, arepas, or biryani. The result is that some kids feel like their food doesn't "count" and, by extension, that *they* don't count either.

"Eat the rainbow" is also often used as a playful challenge to get kids to try more colors. But when it turns into a chart or tracking assignment, it can shift from curiosity to performance. Kids may start focusing on external praise instead of tuning in to their own internal cues.

Purity words like "clean" or "real" imply that processed foods (which many families rely on for cost, access, time, or safety) are "dirty" or less than. The hidden message kids absorb is painful: *My family's food traditions, my body, or my safe foods are wrong.*

Food is never just nutrients. It's memory, identity, connection, and culture. When we erase that, kids are left with judgment instead of joy.

Food Positivity Reframe: All bodies, all foods, all cultures belong at the table.

What You Said	What You Meant	What They Heard	The Hidden Takeaway	Food Positivity Reframe
"Eat the rainbow!"/ "Only clean, real food is good for you."/ "Processed foods are bad."	I want you to eat more fruits and veggies and less packaged food.	My family's food doesn't count. Processed = dirty. Beige/ brown foods are wrong.	My culture, family, or safe foods don't belong. Some bodies and families are better than others.	"Every family has special foods. Eating a variety over time helps our bodies and minds grow strong."

A Note on Nutrition, Health, and Nuance

Two truths can hold at the same time:

- All foods are good foods, and not all foods have the same nutrients.
- All bodies are good bodies, and bodies naturally come in different shapes, sizes, colors, and abilities.

(continued)

(*continued*)

Here's what that means for kids:

- **Different foods do different things:** In your role as the Food Leader, you can guide kids toward enjoying a variety of nourishing foods without teaching fear, secrecy, or guilt. (More on this in Chapter 12.)
- **Nutrition education matters, but timing matters too:** Our job is to meet kids where they are and create learning opportunities that match how they think, feel, and grow.
- **Health is bigger than food:** Stress, access, safety, and care shape well-being, too.
- **Weight stigma harms:** Warnings about size, whether big or small, doesn't improve health. It creates stress and disordered eating.

Bottom line: Food Positivity isn't about skipping the science; it's about broadening it. We look beyond narrow "health-first" lessons and prioritize the Whole-Child. That means teaching about food at the right time, in the right way, starting with curiosity and connection and layering in nuance as kids grow.

Pulling Back the Curtain

Now that you've seen the traps side by side, we can see the bigger picture coming into focus. On the surface they look different—some show up as fear, some as restriction, some as categories or oversimplified claims. But at their core, they share the same pattern: They rely on control. Instead of helping kids listen to their own bodies, they teach kids to follow external rules.

And it's easy to see why catchy phrases, "better categories," or bite-size nutrition lessons feel appealing, especially when they *seem* developmentally aligned. But swapping in nicer sound bites doesn't change the problem. Kids don't need more labels, hierarchies, or rules. They need a completely different way of learning about food, one that honors how they actually think, grow, and make sense of the world and one that protects their natural ability to listen to their bodies.

So at this point, you might be wondering: *What do I say instead? How do I help my kids learn about food without falling into fear, rules, or pressure?*

> Here's the key: It's not about teaching less; it's about teaching better.

"You can't solve a problem with the same thinking that created it."
—Albert Einstein

When we look at the bigger picture—the history, the research, and the cross-disciplinary science—we start to understand that we can't keep using the same solutions and expect different results. That's where the Food Positivity Framework comes in. It gives us a new perspective: one that aligns what kids are ready to learn with *how* we actually teach, through our everyday Modeling, Messaging, and Moments.

Within this framework, the **Learning Foundations** are where your words and actions matter most. Think of them as the conditions that make meaningful food learning possible. They're not scripts to memorize. They're a lens that keeps your child's development, emotions, and sense of belonging at the center of every food conversation.

Guiding Skills = What Parents Practice to Teach

So far, we've looked at the Food Positivity Framework through your child's lens. You understand your Whole-Child at the center, guided by your Family Core Values, and how their Growing Needs and Growing Skills take shape. But you're not just watching from the sidelines. You play a guiding role in helping these skills develop. That's where Guiding Skills come in.

Guiding Skills are the everyday practices you embody. They shape your 3 Ms: how you model, how you talk, and how you create moments of connection. These skills aren't about giving lectures or setting rigid rules. They're about your steady presence and everyday experiences that turn your values into action. When you practice these skills, matching expectations to your child's stage, inviting play and exploration, speaking about food and bodies with respect, you create the kind of environment where trust, curiosity, and confidence can thrive.

The Food Positivity Learning Foundations

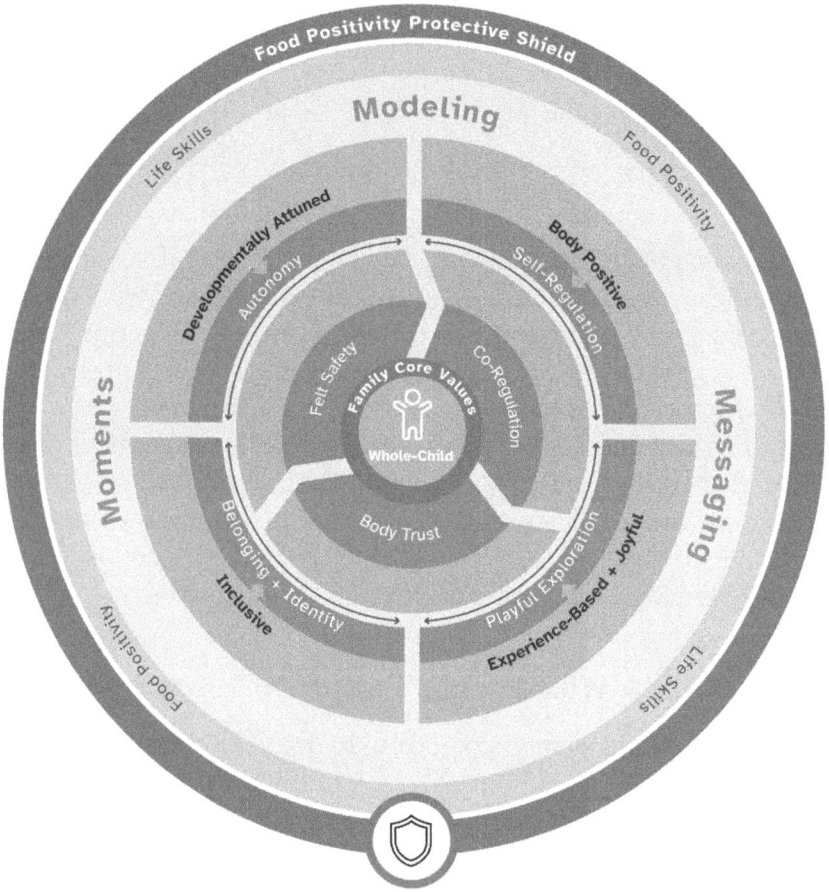

Within the Food Positivity Framework, the Learning Foundations are where Guiding Skills come into focus most clearly. Feeding is the mealtime climate, Environment is the backdrop, and Parenting is the relationship (more on this in Chapter 11!). Learning is about the *how*—the words, examples, and everyday interactions that become your child's food and body lessons and eventually their inner voice.

The Food Talk traps show us what happens when we replace the Guiding Skills with control. The Learning Foundations show us another way: developmentally attuned practices that meet kids where they are and build on their natural curiosity.

Instead of giving kids rigid categories or phrases, the Learning Foundations help you guide with skills that spark exploration, nurture Body Trust, and build resilience against harmful outside messages. They give you a way of teaching that actually matches how kids learn, not how diet culture *wants* them to learn.

Learning Foundations: Guiding Skills (Developmentally Attuned, Body Positive, Experience-Based + Joyful, Inclusive)

Let's focus on the Learning Foundations through your adult perspective. You'll see how each Guiding Skill—Developmentally Attuned, Body Positive, Experience-Based + Joyful, and Inclusive—shows up in daily life and how you can use them with confidence.

Developmentally Attuned (Guiding Skill)

Meet them where they are. Kids think and learn differently at every age and stage.

Being Developmentally Attuned means guiding food learning in ways that fit how your child actually thinks, feels, and grows. It isn't just about choosing the right words; it's about shaping the whole learning experience. The activities you set up, the expectations you hold, even the tone you bring to the table. . .all of it shapes how your child learns about food. When what you teach matches their age and stage, food feels safe, interesting, and engaging. Their brain and body get the message: *Food makes sense to me.*

But, when words and lessons are not aligned with a child's developmental stage, it can be harmful or backfire. A preschooler might take your words literally ("Sugar is poison!") and worry about every extra sprinkle on their cupcake. A teen might roll their eyes at a food rule ("Just eat your veggies") because it feels like you're not respecting their growing autonomy. These mismatches can leave kids confused, anxious, or ashamed because of how they understood it.

When we slow down and match our teaching to how kids actually learn, everything shifts. Food transforms into meaningful experiences that build understanding, trust, and critical thinking. Kids become curious, confident, and connected, and that's what turns food education into Food Positivity.

Everyday Moments That Support Developmental Attunement

- **Early Childhood (2–5):** Sorting fruit by color, shape, or size, reading food-themed storybooks, making tortillas with granny
- **Elementary (6–8):** Looking up "why" questions together, trying simple kitchen science (melting, mixing, freezing), pretending to be food critics and rate tastes
- **Tweens (9–12):** Researching and cooking a recipe from another culture, exploring where food comes from, talking about family food traditions
- **Teens (13–18):** Having real conversations about food marketing and diet culture, exploring how social media affects body image, reflecting on how hunger, fullness, and stress show up for them

When you meet your child where they are, you give them safe choices that build autonomy and feel empowering instead of overwhelming.

Body Positive (Guiding Skill)

Teach through a lens of worth, not rules.

Being Body Positive means teaching kids about food and bodies in ways that affirm their worth, spark curiosity, and celebrate diversity. It's about offering information and experiences that help kids see food as something to explore and bodies as something to respect—in all their shapes, sizes, and rhythms. Their brain and body get the message: *EveryBODY is good. My signals matter. I can regulate from a place of trust, not shame.*

EveryBODY is worthy.
EveryBODY belongs.

When food and body lessons are framed with rules—"That's junk" or "This food gives you quick energy."—kids learn to doubt their cues and compare themselves to others. Instead of staying curious, they shut down, feel judged, or absorb harmful ideas about what makes a body "good."

But when parents model and teach from a Body Positive lens, everything shifts. Food becomes something to discover instead of a test to pass. Bodies become something to celebrate for their differences instead of comparing. Kids learn to question diet culture messages, trust their signals, and take pride in their unique selves.

Everyday Moments That Teach Through a Body Positive Lens

- Celebrating family and cultural food traditions with joy and pride.
- Reading books or pointing out media that show body diversity and challenge narrow beauty ideals.
- Normalizing that everyBODY grows differently, at its own pace, and that's something to celebrate.

When you teach through a Body Positive lens, you give your child space to practice self-regulation, tuning-in to their signals and trusting their body instead of overriding it to meet outside expectations.

Experience-Based + Joyful (Guiding Skill)

Kids learn by doing, not just listening.

Learning about food is full-body, full-senses, and often. . .a "full of crumbs" experience for kids. They learn when they squish their hand in the guacamole bowl and spread it across their tray, when they sniff simmering dal on the stovetop and say, "Mmmmm," or when they press a cookie cutter into dough and proudly shout, "The best cookie spaceship ever!" Those messy, silly, hands-on moments *are* the learning. Their brain and body get the message: *Food is fun. My curiosity belongs here.*

If food always comes with rules—"Don't play with your food" or "Just try one bite"—kids may start to shut down. What looks like "picky eating" or stalling is often just a child's way of saying: *I'm not ready yet. I need more time to explore.*

But when we offer food as something for kids to experience, everything shifts. Kids light up when they get to smush, stack, sort, sniff, stir, and use their imagination. They might turn celery into paintbrushes or treat a spice jar like it's a magic potion. They might pretend with broccoli "trees" for weeks before they ever take a bite and that's part of the journey. That's trust and comfort building underneath each joyful moment.

Everyday Moments That Spark Joyful Learning

- Adding gummy bears to water and watching them expand
- Putting googly eyes on a kohlrabi and pretending it's a baby doll
- Laughing together at food "fails" or funny experiments

When food feels joyful and hands-on, kids get safe chances to explore. That kind of play helps them build comfort and confidence with food.

Inclusive (Guiding Skill)

Everyone deserves to see themselves.

Being inclusive is about creating an environment where your child knows their food, their body, and their traditions are welcome and celebrated. Food is so much more than something we eat; it's memory, comfort, identity, and culture. Being inclusive is a daily practice through the words you choose, the meals you serve, and the way you talk about bodies and cultures. When kids see their preferences respected and their family traditions honored, their brain and body get the message: *Who I am belongs here.*

Kids notice when inclusion is missing. Being teased about a "different" lunch, a casual body comparison, feeling othered when your family's traditional foods are labeled as "unhealthy" in a lesson. All of these things can send the quiet but powerful message that something about them is wrong. Over time, they may start hiding what they eat, feeling embarrassed about their culture, or second-guessing their body.

But when we create an inclusive environment, everything shifts. Kids grow proud of their food and culture and they stay curious about others. They feel safe knowing their body isn't a problem to fix. Inclusion tells them, every single day: *You matter. You belong, exactly as you are.*

Everyday Moments That Support Inclusion

- Skipping negative comments about bodies, sizes, or "weird" foods
- Making space for curiosity about other traditions and cuisines
- Celebrating differences as part of what makes the world rich and meaningful

When you practice inclusion every day, your child feels welcome at the table and grows the deeper life skill of belonging. That sense of worth carries into every part of their world.

Food Exploration: The Gateway to Learning, Connection, and Confidence

Before our kids ever step into a classroom, they're already learning through food—noticing textures, hearing sizzles, smelling herbs, and watching grownups

Food is where life's most meaningful lessons begin.

gather and connect. That first sensory encounter with a banana peel or the squish of the fruit between their fingers? That's learning in motion.

And when we slow down to invite curiosity, something incredible happens: Food becomes so much more than nutrition. It becomes a hands-on, hearts-on, full-body experience where learning comes alive, confidence grows, and relationships deepen. This is food exploration.

What Is Food Exploration?

Food exploration is the foundation of meaningful food learning. It's not about convincing kids to take a bite. It's about giving them space to interact with food in open-ended, developmentally aligned, playful, and fun ways that engage whole-body learning.

It's the swirl of a spoon in a milkshake, the sniff of a cookie baking in the oven, the stacking of crackers into a tower, the belly laugh when an air pocket in refried beans makes a silly noise. These moments might seem small, but they're not. They're the rich, sensory, brain-building bridge between your Guiding Skills and your child's growth.

Food exploration brings the four Learning Foundations to life:

- **Developmentally Attuned:** Meets kids where they are through sensory-rich, concrete experiences that match how they learn.
- **Experience-Based + Joyful:** Hands-on, playful learning that sticks because it's fun.
- **Body Positive:** Builds Body Trust and Autonomy by honoring hunger, fullness, and preferences.
- **Inclusive:** Welcomes all kids, bodies, cultures, and abilities—no moralizing or pressure.

You're not teaching nutrition rules. You're offering an invitation to connect, and that's what kids remember.

For Grown-Ups Wondering, "But What If They Don't Taste It?"

Food exploration asks us to redefine progress.

If your child doesn't taste or even touch a food, it doesn't mean nothing is happening. Every experience sends the message: This food is safe. I get to decide when (or if) I'm ready. That's how we build trust, not with force but with freedom.

Familiarity leads to curiosity. And curiosity? Well, that's what opens the door to trying. . .when they're ready.

Why It Matters

Food exploration builds lifelong skills, from emotional regulation and problem-solving to pattern recognition, vocabulary development, and confidence in navigating the world.

It's naturally cross-disciplinary too. Each moment can invite:

- **Science:** Observing changes when food is cooked or blended
- **Technology:** Using tools or kitchen gadgets
- **Engineering:** Building snack structures or new helpful inventions
- **Art:** Arranging colorful veggies or designing a silly snack face

- **Math:** Measuring, comparing, estimating, dividing
- **History and culture:** Learning family food stories, traditions, and where food comes from

Food isn't just about eating it's about identity, connection, and belonging.

When you slow down and invite food exploration into your daily life, you're not just teaching about food. You're helping your child:

- Build a positive, trusting relationship with their body
- Develop confidence and resilience
- Stay grounded around confusing messages about food and bodies
- Grow into someone who sees food as a source of nourishment and connection

It's not flashy, and it's not a quick fix. But it's real, lasting, and rooted in how children thrive. That's the power of exploration.

Bringing It Home

By now you've seen how easy it is to fall into Food Talk Traps and how common phrases—even the ones meant to help—can send messages kids aren't ready to understand. But at their core, they all share the same pattern: They try to control kids into eating how *we* want them to eat.

Control may bring short-term compliance, but it doesn't build long-term trust. Kids don't need more rules, categories, or clever sound bites. They need food learning that matches how they actually think and grow: simple, concrete, joyful, and connected to their real lives.

The Food Positivity Learning Foundations reimagine food education. It's an evidence-backed way to teach about food through exploration—a safe, playful, and curiosity-driven space where learning and belonging thrive.

And the best part is there is no one-size-fits-all. You just need to stay curious with your child, meet them where they are, and invite them to explore.

Awareness is the first step. Part II helped you see the Invisible Curriculum, understand your child better, and shape a new way to approach food. What follows in Part III will help you start putting everything you learned into practice and raise kids with Food Positivity.

One Simple Step

The next time you feel yourself about to say a "helpful" phrase, take one breath and ask:

"What do I really want my child to learn in this moment?"

Your Food Positivity Practice

Spot & Shift: *Turning Old Food Talk Into New Possibilities*

PART

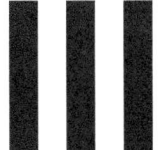

What We're Passing On: Unpacking Diet Culture in Parenting

10

Family Core Values: Shifting Toward a Positive Foundation

I grew up in a home where eating "indulgent" food meant you had no self-control, and my parents constantly worried about how I looked to others. I swore my daughter would never go through that. I want her to enjoy food and love her body. But I struggle with letting her have things like second portions or dessert. I end up feeling guilty about how much she eats, and I can't help worrying what feeding her this way says about me as a parent. Shouldn't I be serving more vegetables? Offering sweets less often? I second-guess every choice.
—Amber

IN PART II, we pulled back the curtain on how kids actually learn about food and bodies. You saw that mealtimes aren't just about eating, they're classrooms where our kids are forming beliefs, wiring their future habits, and learning whether they can trust their bodies. We walked through what kids need at every age and stage, how their brains and bodies process messages, and why they need more than categories or clever phrases to truly eat well. They need us to step outside the same old thinking that created the problem of food rules, body shame, and not having the inner confidence to nourish ourselves well in the first place.

Now, it's time to take action. Let's translate that awareness into change, reshaping the language, routines, and Invisible Curriculum your child experiences at home so they can grow up trusting their body, feeling safe at the table, and enjoying food without guilt.

But before we shift our parenting approach or transform our language, we need to start where everything begins: **your values**.

Looking Back: The Lessons We Inherited

When you take a moment to reflect, you can probably see how the values you grew up shaped you, often in ways you didn't notice at the time. If your parents valued control, obedience, or perfection, you may remember feeling like you never measured up. You may have learned that living up to their standards was the only way to feel worthy, loved, or safe in your own home.

Those experiences may have taught you to doubt your hunger, question your body, and believe that your size or your eating habits determined your worth. And they echo into adulthood, not only in your struggles to feed your child but also as self-doubt, the pressure to achieve, and the feeling that no matter what you do, it's never quite enough.

Your parents didn't set out to harm you. They relied on the tools they had, shaped by the culture they grew up in themselves. And even if you didn't grow up with strict, controlling values, it's worth noticing how diet culture (and its crafty siblings, purity and hustle culture) pushes these values into our daily lives—through social media, medical advice, work and school culture, and even casual conversations with friends and family.

Over time, all of these messages became part of *your* Invisible Curriculum, quietly shaping how you came to think about food, your body, and your place in the world. But when we pause to name what we inherited, we can loosen its grip. We gain self-compassion and create space to choose a different path for our kids—one built on values that support Food Positivity.

Parent Reflection

You've made it this far, and maybe things are starting to click. You're beginning to see not only how kids grow and learn but also how diet culture shaped *your* story and how it still shows up at your table.

That realization can be freeing, but it can also stir up grief. You might find yourself thinking about what could have been different for you, if only *you* had been parented in this way.

That's part of this process, difficult as it is. And it's also okay to feel unsure about what comes next. The good news is you don't need to have been parented this way to pass a better story on to your kids. Our own parents did the best they could with what they knew. Now you have tools and knowledge they didn't. And with them, the chance to choose a different way forward.

Taking a Critical Look at the Negative Values You Grew Up With

The following are common values tied to the restrictive and controlling style of parenting. Some of these values may have supported you, but many likely got in the way of feeling safe with food, trusting your body, or exploring food with curiosity rather than fear. It's not a complete list, but naming them can help you see what you've been carrying and begin to decide which ones you're ready to let go.

Negative Values + Beliefs

Control Rules were used to show who's in charge and keep those with less power in line. As a child, your success depended on following those rules, with little room for your personal needs, questions, or individuality.

Obedience Safety felt possible only when you did as you were told. Fear of consequences, whether for how you behaved, what you ate, how you looked, or even when you expressed your feelings, taught us that acceptance depended on constant compliance.

Conformity Outside standards decided what was "good" or "acceptable." Your belonging depended on fitting into narrow ideals, not just about body size and eating patterns but often things like your sexuality or career path too. Going against these norms meant risking judgment and exclusion.

Self-Sacrifice   Your worth was measured by how much you carried, how hard you worked, and what you gave up—even if it left you exhausted. Your productivity and self-denial were more valuable than your needs for rest, joy, and satisfaction, teaching you that saying "yes" to everyone else mattered more than taking care of yourself.

Achievement   Feeling accepted depended on proving yourself. Success—usually defined by someone else's standards—was the only way to gain respect, whether through the body size you achieved, academics, or anything else.

Perfection   Your worth depended on getting everything "right," including how you looked, behaved, and represented your family. The pressure to be perfect left little room for fun, mistakes, or play, and likely contributed to rigid behaviors.

Healthism   Health—or at least the appearance of it—was a personal obligation and badge of virtue. Instead of supporting your well-being, it was about living up to a predetermined "picture" of health to prove your discipline and avoid the judgment of others.

What's So Wrong with Wanting to Be Healthy?

In short, absolutely nothing. Prioritizing your family's health is an incredible thing! When we talk about "healthism" as a negative, control-oriented value, we don't mean there's anything wrong with making choices that genuinely support your health.

The trouble with the value of healthism is that it turns choosing a predefined set of "healthy" behaviors into a performance, often pushing us toward actions that don't *actually* support our needs, like eating too little, overexercising, or denying ourselves foods we enjoy.

So please, offer vegetables or go on that family bike ride—or whatever choices fit *your* family best. The point isn't the specific activity; it's the intention behind it. Do it because it truly supports your family's well-being, not because you feel pressured to meet someone else's version of "healthy."

Choosing the Values You Want Your Kids to Grow Up With

You want your child's story with food and their body to be different. And yet, it's deeply human to hold onto the messages you grew up with. On some level, those old lessons felt like safety, even if they ultimately caused you harm.

But the truth is, if the choices we make as parents are still rooted in that same fear and control, nothing really changes. When we parent from these inherited values, we unintentionally work against the very needs we explored in Part II. You may swap harsh words for gentler ones, but the result is the same: a home environment that teaches control, not trust.

The diet culture promise—that if you just say the right thing, teaching them the "right" lessons about nutrition, your child will eat "well" and grow into an "acceptable" body—it just doesn't work. It's the same old story dressed up in a shiny new wrapper, and it only reinforces the same harm.

Crafting something truly supportive means pausing to question what we inherited and choosing to act from an entirely different set of values. Let's take a look at the kinds of positive values and beliefs that help our kids thrive.

> *Your values aren't just words; they're the compass your child uses to navigate food and body messages for the rest of their life.*

Positive Values + Beliefs

Supportive Leadership   Being a supportive parent and Food Leader means stepping into your role with steadiness and care, not control. You set the structure—like serving meals at predictable times, including at least one safe food, and gently offering new foods without pressure—so your child knows what to count on (*Felt Safety*). At the same time, you trust their signals and respect their pace, creating room for curiosity, comfort, and growth (*Autonomy*, *Playful Exploration*). Supportive leadership guides kids as they grow and helps them become confident, capable adults.

Safety   Kids thrive when they feel safe, both physically and emotionally. You consistently provide enough food for your child to grow and remove pressure, shame, and rigid rules so your kids can relax, explore, and trust that both their body and their needs will be cared for (*Felt Safety* + *Body Trust*). And when it comes to literal safety, you support your child through navigating harmful food and body messages and manage real food-related risks like allergies, choking hazards, and nutrition deficiencies.

Agency   Agency is about choice and dignity. You offer options within your supportive boundaries and respect your child's hunger, fullness, and preferences (*Autonomy*). You also invite their preferences into your family's food culture, like regularly serving what they enjoy. These small moments teach kids that their voice matters and they can trust their bodies, supporting self-confidence and decision-making skills far beyond the table (*Self-Regulation*, *Body Trust*).

Individuality   Every child is unique in body size, shape, sensory needs, and eating style. Some kids love crunchy foods while others prefer soft; some kids need lots of food while others need less. Valuing individuality means you celebrate differences instead of trying to make every child (or every plate) look the same. You model that all bodies are worthy of care and dignity, and you help kids build confidence in who they are (*Belonging* + *Identity*). Making space for curiosity and flexibility shows your child that their choices matter and that they have the freedom to engage with food and their body in ways that fit their unique self (*Autonomy*).

Connection   Food is more than fuel; it's one of the most powerful ways we connect with each other. Connection is about slowing down to share meals when you can, being emotionally present, and noticing when your child needs comfort or play more than a perfect diet (*Co-Regulation*). This deep bond between you and your child is the foundation for growth. When kids feel connected, they feel seen—and that sense of belonging helps them feel safe to be themselves and try new things (*Belonging* + *Identity*, *Playful Exploration*).

Joy and Wonder   Kids learn best when food is fun. These moments might look like giggling over watermelon juice running down your chin, savoring Grandma's soup, or experimenting with a new recipe together. Joy makes food pleasurable, and wonder helps kids feel curious to keep exploring (*Playful Exploration*). Together, they make food something kids *want* to explore, not just something they're supposed to eat. When you make room for joy and wonder, you show your child that food is not only about fueling their body but also about celebrating life (*Belonging + Identity*).

Well-Being   True health and well-being is about the whole person. It includes physical, mental, emotional, and social health, as well as trust in your own body—not just how you look, eat, or the number on your scale. You model this by caring for your body with compassion and by acknowledging the bigger picture influencing health, including food access, stress, and community. And all the while, you encourage balanced, flexible habits that feel good and last (*Felt Safety, Autonomy, Self-Regulation*).

Keep in mind that this list is designed to give you some general direction, but you might choose alternative words like **autonomy, belonging, curiosity, kindness, flexibility, trust, identity**, or **respect**.

Most of those words fit somewhere within the core values we've named, but each family can decide which words feel right for them and shape their list in a way that reflects what matters most in their home.

Sorting Through the Values Trauma Left Behind

When we've grown up with trauma, re-examining our values can feel unsettling. The beliefs you once held were survival tools that kept you safe in an environment where your needs weren't respected. Maybe you learned that obedience was the only way to stay safe or that self-sacrifice was how you kept the peace.

(continued)

(*continued*)

As a child, those strategies made sense and helped you get through hard moments. But as an adult, and especially as a parent, you're now faced with the question: *Do these old rules still serve me?*

Letting go of survival-based values can feel scary, even like betraying your family or the younger version of yourself who relied on them. But re-evaluating your values isn't about erasing your past; it's about choosing what you want to carry forward and what no longer has a place in your life or your child's.

If this feels heavy or confusing, you don't have to navigate it alone. A trauma-informed therapist or dietitian can be *your* safe guide as you recognize patterns, grieve what you didn't receive, and choose values that reflect the parent you want to be today.

Reframing Fear-Driven Parenting into Value-Driven Parenting

Yet even when we know that values like agency, safety, and individuality are a better path forward for our kids, it's still hard work to keep the fears diet culture has planted so deep inside us from creeping back in. They show up as a little voice in our heads: *"If I let them eat that, I'm failing,"* or *"If I don't make them finish, they'll never learn."*

But this is exactly how diet culture keeps us stuck. Out of fear, we make reactive choices that don't align with what we really want our kids to learn. But with practice, we can stop these fears in their tracks and re-frame them to align with our new values. Here's how those fears might sound and how you can reframe your response:

Situation	Fear-Based Thought	Value-Driven Reframe
Child asks for chips after school	*Healthism:* "If I let them eat chips, they'll become unhealthy, and I'll fail at keeping them well."	*Well-being:* "Chips can be part of a balanced pattern. Allowing enjoyment supports trust, satisfaction, and overall well-being."

Situation	Fear-Based Thought	Value-Driven Reframe
Child's body is larger than their peers'	*Conformity:* "If my child doesn't lose weight, others will judge me, and they'll struggle socially."	*Individuality:* "Bodies come in different sizes. Supporting my child's individuality and body trust will help them feel safe and confident."
Child leaves vegetables on their plate	*Obedience:* "If I don't make them finish, they may never learn to eat vegetables."	*Safety:* "Trusting my child to listen to their body keeps eating safe and respectful. I can keep offering vegetables without pressure."

When Your Co-Parent Isn't Ready for Change

Putting these value-driven reframes into practice is hard work on its own, but it's even harder if your co-parent isn't ready to move away from fear-based thinking or doesn't yet see the need for change.

It might feel like your co-parent is willing to let harm come to your child, but that's rarely the full story. Parents often come to the table with different beliefs, shaped by their own childhoods, cultural backgrounds, and experiences with diet culture. One may have faced more harm—because of body size, gender, neurodivergence, or any other privilege they don't hold—and be more motivated to prevent it for their child. The other may not share those experiences or may still be desperately seeking the sense of safety or acceptance that diet culture promises.

Try to connect around the goals you already share: raising kids who are healthy, happy, and safe. Where you disagree is probably the exact process of how to get there. Focusing on that bigger picture leaves space for your values to align over time. (We'll share a resource to help with this in Chapter 12.)

And even if you're the only one leading the change, your influence matters. Each time you act from supportive values, your child feels it. Over time, your steady example can have a lasting impact, even if your co-parent isn't ready to join you yet.

The Hard Truth About Size and Safety

A sad but true reality is that as long as the world is steeped in diet culture, thinness *does* come with a kind of safety. Parents aren't wrong to worry that a child in a larger body may face teasing, bullying, medical bias, or discrimination later in life. But encouraging a child to shrink their body promotes shame and disordered eating, which doesn't keep them safe either.

This puts parents of kids in larger bodies who truly value safety in an awful position. And if you've lived in a larger body yourself, you may feel that fear deep in your body, because you know exactly how painful it can be.

There's a word for a system that keeps people from meeting their essential needs: *oppression.* And if you still feel uncertain about the right move, know that it's not a flaw in your parenting. It's the natural tension of wanting the best for your child in a world that isn't designed to support them.

We can't end an oppressive system overnight, but we can give kids tools to navigate it. We can affirm that their bodies are perfect just as they are, create homes where their needs are truly met, and equip them with the skills to resist and challenge oppression right alongside us.

Individual Family Values + Beliefs

Beyond the overall positive values and beliefs that support everyone thriving, your family will also have values that are uniquely yours. Your individual values are shaped by your experiences, what *you* believe matters most, and what you want to pass on to your children.

There's no single "right" way to approach this work. What one family feels is as a must-have, another might see as not useful at all. In fact, a lot of the tension in parenting spaces (often called the "mommy wars") happens when we treat our individual values like rules everyone else should follow. That pulls us right back into control and comparison, which is the opposite of what we want to model for our kids.

So use the following sections as inspiration, not a prescription. Notice which ones feel like "yes, that's us," which ones feel like "not for us right now," and which ones spark curiosity or conversation with your co-parent or support system.

Cultural and Religious Traditions

Food can be a way to celebrate who you are and where you come from. Cooking a recipe passed down through generations, observing religious food practices (like kosher or halal), or sharing a special holiday meal teaches kids that food is part of your family's story.

Community and Social Justice

Maybe your family expresses its values through supporting local farmers, choosing products with fair labor practices, or advocating for better food access in your community. This shows children that food is part of a bigger system and that they have the power to make a difference.

Environmental Stewardship

For some families, food choices are a way of caring for the planet—like buying sustainably grown produce, reducing food waste, or enjoying more plant-forward meals. This teaches kids that what we eat connects to the earth we all share.

Animal Welfare

Some families prioritize reducing or eliminating animal products or sourcing food from farms that follow humane practices. These choices show children that compassion and ethics can guide what goes on their plate.

Practical Convenience

Sometimes the most nourishing choice is the easiest one. Serving frozen meals, prechopped produce, or takeout can free up time and energy for connection, rest, or simply a calmer evening. Choosing convenience is not "lazy"—it's a valid way to support your family's well-being.

Financial Stewardship

For many families, following a budget and living within their means is important. Planning meals, cooking at home, or creatively stretching ingredients helps balance nourishment with financial stability. These practices save money without turning home cooking into a judgment of being "better" than other options.

Mindfulness

Some families focus on noticing the current moment and reflecting on how their meals provide nourishment and satisfaction. This might look like pausing for a moment of thanks before eating or talking about what everyone is grateful for at the table.

Generosity and Hospitality

Food can also be a way to care for others, like hosting friends, sharing meals with neighbors, or cooking for someone who's sick. These experiences teach children that food connects us and that sharing what we have builds community.

> **EXPERT INSIGHT: Balancing Personal Values + Agency: A Vegan Mom's Perspective**
>
> Taylor Wolfram, RDN, of Taylor Wolfram Nutrition Counseling and @taylorwolframrd
>
> As a vegan mom and anti-diet registered dietitian, I know what it's like to walk the line of instilling your family values in your kids while also fostering a sense of autonomy and body trust.

I view animal liberation as a part of body liberation, and the values of compassion, respect, and justice for all are ones that I am teaching my kids. While my kids are still quite young, they know that we don't eat animals because we love them and don't want to hurt them.

I know that one day they will gain more independence with food when they're in the school cafeteria and social settings. My hope is that they make choices that align with these values, while also feeling free to experiment and explore as needed for their own sense of agency. I know that forcing, shaming, or punishing is not helpful, and I never want them to feel like they have to hide their food choices from me for fear of judgment. My wish is for them to maintain their veganism if it's what they want to do and it's what feels aligned for them, not because they feel like they have to.

Building Your Framework Foundations: Family Core Values

Now that we've examined the types of values that support Food Positivity in your home, it's time to bring it all together. This is where your Family Core Values come in—the foundation we first mentioned in Chapter 5.

Think of your Family Core Values like a recipe with two key ingredients: the positive values and beliefs that support every child's growth and the individual ones that reflect your family's unique story. When you mix those together, you create Core Values that are yours alone— your family's special recipe.

There's no "right" list of Core Values and no one-size-fits-all formula. And your Core Values may grow and evolve over time right along with your family. What matters is that your kids hear clear, supportive messages again and again.

A Note on Guilt

The phrase "guilt and shame" comes up often when we talk about breaking cycles and building something better for our kids. Our goal is to help you feed without either—but they're not synonyms.

Shame is the belief that we are inherently bad, because of our body size, eating preferences, or any other natural part of who we are. And it has no place in feeding or parenting. Guilt, on the other hand, is the feeling that arises when our actions don't line up with our values.

As you work on living out your Family Core Values, you can use guilt to your advantage. When it comes knocking, ask yourself: "Is this feeling because I'm trying to live out positive values, but my beliefs are still rooted in negative ones?" If the answer is yes, let your guilt be a gentle signal that it's time to pause and realign with the values you truly want to carry forward.

Core Values in Action: The 3 Ms

As we explored in Chapter 7, these repeated messages—the Modeling, Messaging, and Moments your child experiences—form the backbone of the Invisible Curriculum that supports your child as they build Food Positivity. And what drives those 3 Ms is your values.

When we're drawing on negative, fear-based values like control and obedience, the Invisible Curriculum ends up teaching shame and body distrust. But that's what makes the 3 Ms so powerful—because when they're grounded in *positive* Family Core Values, they communicate trust, care, and belonging instead.

The clearer you are on your values, the more you'll be able to use the 3 Ms for good. Let's take a look at how the 3 Ms differ depending on the values driving our actions and what our kids learn as a result.

Situation	Parent Response (Value)	Child Learns
Shopping for new clothes (Moments)	"Let's find something more flattering to hide your stomach." (*conformity*)	"My body is wrong. I have to dress to make it acceptable."
	"Let's find clothes you feel comfortable and confident in." (*individuality*)	"I can show my body just as it is. It's okay to be different. What matters is how I feel and that my style expresses what I want."
Family eating dinner together (Messaging)	"You finished all your vegetables, good job!" (*achievement*)	"I'm worthy when I perform and meet expectations."
	"I love how we all sat and talked together at dinner." (*connection*)	"What matters most is being together."
Brownies for dessert (Modeling)	"No brownies for me! I've got to stay on track with my diet." (*perfection*)	"Eating dessert means losing control or failing. To be 'good,' I'll need to deny myself like my parent does."
	"These brownies look delicious! I'm glad we made them and get to enjoy them together." (*joy & wonder*)	"Sharing food is about connection and pleasure."

A Protective Shield Against Diet Culture

Once you've identified your Core Values and you are regularly living them out through the 3 Ms, they become part of your child's Protective Shield, strengthening their resilience against diet culture and helping them feel safe and confident in their own body.

This shield won't block every outside message, but it acts like a filter, helping your child pause, sort through the noise, and decide what to take in—and what to leave behind.

Living in a home driven by your Family Core Values doesn't guarantee your child will never struggle with food or body image. But it gives them something powerful to return to:

Over time, this foundation becomes an inner compass—your child's north star—that they can rely on in tough moments, giving them the confidence to step into the world with clarity, resilience, and trust in themselves.

Bringing It Home

The values you carry—whether inherited or chosen—are at the core of the decisions you make about food, bodies, and everything else. You may have grown up with control, obedience, or perfection as guiding forces, and it's natural for those values to surface in your parenting now. But by identifying those old, harmful patterns, you create space to pause, reflect, and choose what you truly want to pass on.

As your child moves through new stages of life—friendships, school, adolescence, and beyond—they will return again and again to the foundation your Family Core Values have built. A home grounded in values like safety, connection, and true well-being will give them the confidence to make choices that feel right for *them*, even when outside pressures push them in another direction (much more on this in Chapter 19).

And you're growing too. The more you live out your Family Core Values, the more you'll be able to step into being the kind of parent and Food Leader you want to be. Your values are not just lessons you're teaching but the steady ground *you* stand on—guiding your family through tough decisions, celebrations, discoveries, and the everyday rhythms that shape your life together.

One Simple Step

The next time a food or body situation comes up with your child, pause and ask yourself: "Where's this coming from?" Try to name the value behind your thoughts or actions. Noticing the root of your reaction is the first step toward change.

Your Food Positivity Practice

Creating Our Family Core Values: *Choosing What Matters Most*

11

Parenting Matters: Guiding with Confidence and Care

Before I became a parent, I never imagined I could get so angry about something as simple as dinner. But when my son refuses to eat, I can't help but snap over how rude it is to not even try the food I spent time cooking. He'll push the plate away and whine for something else. Most nights, he eats almost nothing, and I'm left wondering why his behavior sets me off so much.

—Anthony

EVEN WITH STRONG Family Core Values in place in your home, children can't navigate food and body experiences on their own. They're still learning to listen to what their bodies are communicating, manage big feelings, and understand themselves in the world, both with food and beyond.

Your values help guide your choices, but your parenting approach is the way you live them out each day, helping your child build the skills to eat well and trust themselves. And it isn't about following any one parenting approach to the letter. What matters are the small, intentional practices you carry out, day after day, as you show up for your child.

It's the way you shape their environment, offer rhythms they can count on, and step in with support when the situations are confusing or overwhelming. These tasks are a central part of your role as the Food Leader. You're not just putting meals on the table; you're creating the conditions for your child to do their part too by actively meeting their Growing Needs as they learn to listen, explore, and trust themselves.

This partnership is at the heart of Food Positivity. And far from being just a hopeful idea, this balance reflects a well-established, evidence-based approach to parenting and feeding kids—one that connects the values you hold with the everyday choices and interactions that bring them to life.

So let's explore how parenting styles shape children's experiences—and how your Guiding Needs are the tools that turn your Family Core Values into lived experiences at the table.

Your Parenting Style Matters

Parenting researchers often describe four main types of parenting styles that differ based on two elements: warmth and structure. Warmth is the love, encouragement, and responsiveness (noticing your child's cues and showing up with care) that helps kids feel valued and connected. Structure is the guidance, routines, and boundaries that give kids a sense of safety and predictability. How much warmth and structure we bring to our parenting approaches influence everything from emotional development to eating behaviors.

When we look at these parenting styles through a food parenting lens, we find that most parents don't fit neatly into just one style. When you read the following table, you may see yourself in more than one depending on the day, your child, or even how stressed you feel.

High Structure

Low warmth			High warmth

Authoritarian ("Because I said so") Parent sets strict rules and expects obedience and allows little or no input from the child. **Example:** Dinner includes only foods the parent approves of. Parent says, "No, dessert unless you finish all your vegetables."	**Authoritative** ("Love with limits") Parent sets clear expectations but listens, supports, and allows kids appropriate choices. **Example:** Dinner is served family-style with options including a safe food. Parent says, "Eat what feels right for your body, today."
Neglectful/Uninvolved ("On your own") Parent is disengaged, often because of stress or other struggles, so kids lack guidance and support. **Example:** Parent doesn't notice the child hasn't eaten. Food is available but without encouragement or connection.	**Permissive** ("Child drives decisions") Parent avoids limits and lets the child take the lead, often to keep the peace. **Example:** Child refuses the meal. Parent quickly offers alternatives: "Okay, I'll make you mac and cheese instead."

Low Structure

Research shows that kids do best when parents lean toward an **authoritative** style of parenting that balances warmth and structure. This approach helps children build trust, practice self-regulation, and develop resilience against outside pressures. Authoritative parenting also supports overall well-being, while authoritarian parenting is linked to poorer self-regulation, higher levels of anxiety and depression, and lower overall self-esteem.

When kids grow up under authoritarian control, they often become more vulnerable to outside pressures—hello, diet culture!—because they haven't learned to trust their own abilities. Permissive and neglectful parenting styles also fall short because without both warmth and structure, kids miss the support and guidance they need to feel safe and grow. These three approaches are linked to difficulties with self-regulation and emotional well-being, since they don't provide children the steady care they need to thrive.

You may recognize in your own story how controlling values—or even the absence of a clear value system—shaped the way your parents approached feeding and parenting. And when the parenting *you* were raised with didn't offer the kind of support children actually need, stepping into that role for your child is certainly a challenge.

Responsive Parenting Includes Responsive Feeding

These parenting styles help us understand the role of warmth and structure in shaping how our parenting approach influences our kids. But even authoritative parenting *can* be applied in ways that center the *parent's* goals, often asking the question, "What parenting strategies produce the best behavior?" Newer parenting models build on the benefits of authoritative parenting but also center the child's development, asking "What strategies equip children with the skills they need to thrive?" This is where responsive parenting comes in.

Variations on responsive parenting have names you might recognize: *respectful*, *gentle*, *attachment-based*, and *conscious* are all popular, especially with parents looking to break the cycle of controlling or hands-off parenting they grew up with themselves. Though the terminology varies, they all emphasize emotional awareness, mutual respect, and honoring the child's individuality.

Research shows these approaches support many of the same benefits we see with authoritative parenting, plus give the child strong emotional regulation skills and a deep sense of connection with their families. And at the heart of all these models is a parent who shows up as a steady, thoughtful leader with the child's best interest always in mind—someone who offers guidance when it's needed most, before a child has the skills to make those decisions on their own.

When applied to how we feed our kids, this approach has been studied under the term *responsive feeding*. Research beginning in the 2010s shows that responsive feeding is associated with greater food variety, stronger recognition of hunger and fullness cues, and a lower risk of disordered eating later in life.

Within the responsive approach, a caregiver's feeding responsibilities are to:

- Create an enjoyable mealtime environment with comfortable seating, clear expectations, and appropriate, appealing foods served on a predictable schedule
- Monitor and support the child's hunger and satiety (fullness) cues
- Respond to the child's feeding cues promptly, with emotional support, and in a way that is developmentally appropriate and aligned with the child's unique needs

If that sounds a lot like what we're after with Food Positivity, you're right! As you know, our aim isn't perfect nutrition at every meal. It's raising children with the confidence and self-regulation to fuel their bodies well over time.

Guiding Needs = What Parents Need to Show Up Well

Now let's shift from theory to practice. With your Whole-Child at the center and your Family Core Values to lean on, it's time to meet your child's Growing Needs with your own Guiding Needs.

These are the mindsets and emotional anchors that help you stay calm, steady, and tuned-in. When you're grounded, you create the safe, consistent environment your child depends on. Some days that comes easily; other days it takes work. That's just real life.

What helps is paying attention—noticing your own stress, hunger, or triggers, and making small shifts: pausing before reacting, reminding yourself of your values, or taking a breath. Every time you steady yourself, you give your child the safety they need to keep growing.

The Food Positivity Parenting Foundations

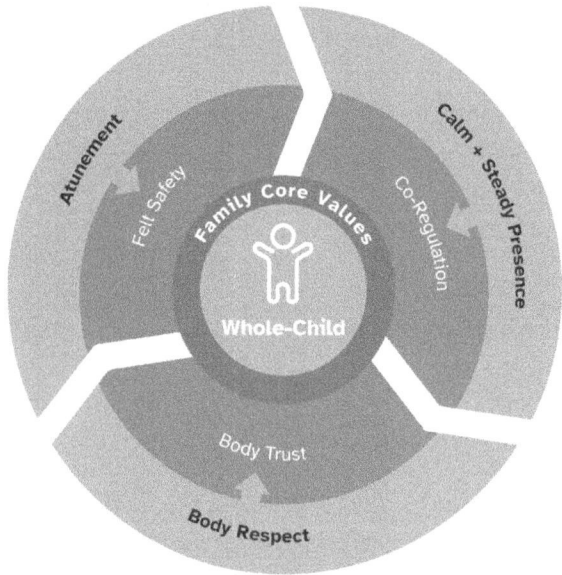

Guiding Needs are the foundation for how you show up as a parent, responsive to your child's needs. If this sounds good in theory but hard in practice, you're not alone. For many of us, the hardest part isn't believing in the benefits of responsive feeding; it's figuring out how to notice and respond to our child's cues when we didn't always have parents who could notice and respond to ours.

Those tantrums or meltdowns that you now recognize as development and a "brain under construction" are the cues; that's them telling you their Growing Needs.

The Food Positivity Parenting Foundations are here to help you recognize those cues and respond in supportive ways so your child can practice their Growing Skills inside a safe, trusting, connected feeding relationship.

Parenting Foundations: Guiding Needs (Attunement, Calm + Steady Presence, Body Respect)

These three Guiding Needs shape how you show up in moments that matter most, supporting your capacity to respond with connection, steadiness, and respect.

Attunement (Guiding Need)

Kids feel safe when they feel understood.

If you've ever rolled your eyes because your child wanted their sandwich cut in a different way or insisted that they stay seated at the table when they might really need to get their wiggles out, those were opportunities for Attunement.

Don't worry—it's very human to be frustrated in these moments! But these are the ways your child expresses that they need you to meet their need for Felt Safety. Attunement is your ability to notice and respond to your child's unique cues—both physical and emotional—in ways that show them the world is predictable and they can trust you to notice what matters to them.

Importantly, Felt Safety looks different for every child. One might not mind if the foods on their plate touch, while another feels safest when you take care to serve each component separately. And you know your child better than anyone else.

When you responded to your child's cries as an infant, that was attunement. It just gets trickier as our children grow, because we start layering in expectations: *Use your words. Take three bites. Don't be so picky.*

Expectations are a good thing when they're developmentally aligned, like asking a preschooler to use kind words or wait 10 minutes for a snack. But often, our expectations are shaped by diet culture. We expect our children to eat and grow a certain way, and we feel pressure to "fix it" if they don't. And when we focus too much on what *should* be happening, we risk missing the connection our kids actually need.

But when you adjust your child's environment, your expectations, or your own presence to meet your child where they are through attunement, everything shifts. You show them, *I see you. I understand what helps you feel safe and I'm here to help.* Your child learns they don't need to fight or hide to feel safe exactly as they are, paving the way for Autonomy and Belonging + Identity.

Everyday Moments That Demonstrate Attunement:

- Remembering details that matter, like the pasta shape your child likes best
- Planning meals for the times your child is naturally most hungry
- Buying foods your child shows interest in, even if they're not part of your norm

Critics of attuned parenting often say these practices "coddle" kids. But Attunement isn't only about meeting needs—it's also about knowing when your child is ready for a gentle challenge. These are the small nudges that help them build new skills as they grow.

Everyday Moments That Challenge with Attunement:

- Ordering a different kind of chicken nuggets at a restaurant when their usual isn't available, trusting that they have the skills to manage the difference
- Gently holding the boundary that you're not serving more food, because they refused their typical bedtime snack are asking to delay bedtime
- Serving a mixed dish instead of separating ingredients, after seeing they've handled similar combinations

Not every child will be ready for these challenges, and that's okay. Neither of these lists consists of things you should always do, but they're examples of attuned decisions you might make depending on what you feel is the right accommodation—or challenge—for your child in the moment. Just like taking the training wheels off a bike, there's no "correct" time to do it. Your job is to notice when they might be ready and provide just the right challenge to help them grow.

And some kids, including those with ARFID, autism, and other specific feeding challenges may not ever be ready for these types of challenges, and that's okay too (more on supporting kids with feeding differences in Chapter 13).

That said, no parent gets attunement right all the time. And you don't need to. What matters is being responsive often enough that your child knows they can count on you. When you miss a cue, coming back with curiosity and care can actually strengthen the trust between you. Repair shows your child that their needs still matter, even if you weren't able to meet them right away.

When Attunement Feels Hard

Over time, the Felt Safety you foster for your child through Attunement strengthens the trust between you. Your child learns that their needs matter, they can go at their own pace, and they won't be forced into someone else's standards. This helps them feel safe to try new things, develop resilience, and build confidence around food and in so many other parts of life.

If you grew up with parents who dismissed or couldn't meet your needs, learning to notice and respond to your child's cues may take time and practice. And if it feels foreign, that doesn't mean you're failing. It means you're doing the brave work of breaking a cycle. And by staying curious instead of judgmental, you may even find yourself more able to notice and honor what you need to feel safe—a skill many of us never had modeled but can reclaim now.

EXPERT INSIGHT: Supporting Felt Safety with Foster Kids

Laura, Founder of Foster Parent Partner @foster.parenting

Disclosure: *This insight is not professional advice. It reflects the lived experience of thousands of foster caregivers and community members who have shared how they support kids in their homes.*

(continued)

(*continued*)

Helping Kids Feel Safe

For caregivers stepping in during a traumatic time in a child's life, tuning into a child's needs and helping them feel safe may require extra patience and additional steps. Kids who have experienced food insecurity or food-related trauma (such as having meals withheld as punishment) may not immediately feel safe in the home.

It can take days, weeks, or months for a child to feel secure and for caregivers to understand their needs as it relates to feeding. Because of this, caregivers often find that focusing on small, day-to-day moments can make the biggest difference in building connection and trust.

Strategies That Build Connection and Trust

- **Offer choice and control.** Their world has been turned upside down, so inviting snack and meal choices can help them regain a sense of control.
- **Stick to a consistent meal and snack schedule.** Over time, kids may feel less worried about when or whether their next meal will come.
- **Keep a stocked fridge at all times.** A full, visible fridge can reassure kids that there will always be food available here.
- **Provide "anytime" snacks.** Keep a selection of snacks in a basket or dedicated fridge bin that kids can access freely.
- **Create safe storage.** Give kids a special spot, like a mini fridge, sealed containers, or a pantry bin, for food that belongs just to them and that they can store themselves. Ensuring that food is "safe" and can't be eaten by anyone else in the home may decrease the likelihood of kids hiding food in their rooms.

When to Seek Professional Support

If you have concerns about a child's eating habits, growth, or health, connect with pediatricians, dietitians, or feeding specialists for additional support.

Calm + Steady Presence (Guiding Need)

Regulation starts with our steadiness.

If you've ever caved to your child's pleas for candy just to stop the whining or snapped in frustration when they didn't touch their dinner, let us assure you. . .you are a very normal parent! But these are examples of a parent who is *not* demonstrating the calm and steady presence children need to work through their big feelings about food.

Co-Regulation is your child's need for someone to support them through the things they can't manage on their own yet. Your Calm + Steady Presence is how you provide it. Children are born with the ability to sense hunger and fullness, but not with the ability to regulate emotions or make logical decisions about feeding. So when you show up with grounded, steady energy, you help them navigate their big feelings and slowly build their own capacity to regulate.

When parents respond to their kids' struggles with anger or frustration, kids learn that their needs aren't safe to express. They may shut down or override their hunger signals to avoid conflict, escalate mealtime battles in a desperate attempt to be heard, or turn to sneaking food to meet their needs. Just giving your child what they want doesn't help either, because it leaves kids without the guidance they need to work through challenging situations. Over time, these patterns can turn into adults who suppress their needs and struggle to make balanced choices.

But when you bring your Calm + Steady Presence, everything shifts. Your child can show up exactly as they are: imperfect and learning. Your ability to calmly guide your child through their feelings—both emotional and physical—helps them build the skills they'll carry forward into Self-Regulation. This opens the door to Body Trust and shows them their needs are worth honoring.

Everyday Moments That Demonstrate Your Calm + Steady Presence

- Acknowledging their feelings about food without judgment ("I hear you're upset about what's for dinner")
- Responding calmly to food refusal and directing your child to other options
- Supporting and empathizing with your child when they feel uncomfortable after overeating

When Your Calm + Steady Presence Feels Hard

If no one guided you through your feelings as a child, it makes sense that regulation—both physical and emotional—doesn't come naturally now. You may find yourself yelling, shutting down, or over-pleasing just to get through emotional challenges, not to mention how difficult it is to navigate your body's sensations.

Still, as your child's grown-up, you have the opportunity to support these skills in your child, beginning with how you nurture them in yourself. By practicing tools like mindfulness and self-compassion, you strengthen your ability to pause, choose your response, and stay present even during stressful times. And each time you pause instead of react, or extend compassion instead of criticism, you build a new pattern—for your kids and for yourself.

Bonus Handout via the QR Code: Becoming the Steady Guide Your Child Needs

Your child's need for Co-Regulation and your Calm + Steady Presence go hand in hand. When you meet in this way, you're not just getting through mealtime struggles, you're nurturing safety, trust, and resilience that will last a lifetime.

Body Respect (Guiding Need)

Kids trust themselves when we respect them.

If you've ever urged your child to take a few more bites after they said they were full or quietly served smaller portions out of fear they might gain weight, know that these are common responses shaped by diet culture. They don't support the Body Trust your child truly needs to care for their body and feel confident in their cues.

Body Respect is your role in making that trust possible. It means honoring your child's body—their size, appetite, preferences, and unique needs. When you consistently show respect for their body, you reinforce the message that their signals matter and their body is inherently worthy of care.

Kids pick up quickly when we think something about them isn't "right." If they sense that your approval depends on eating differently, looking different, or wanting the "right" foods, they learn to ignore their own cues and shape themselves to meet outside expectations. Over time, this can lead to shame about their appetites and bodies, disconnection from hunger and fullness cues, and difficulty trusting their needs.

In feeding, Body Respect means listening to your child's hunger and fullness cues, honoring their pace with food, and respecting their right to say "no," even when you'd rather they say "yes." It's creating an environment where their input matters and they're never pressured to change who they are.

When parents consistently practice Body Respect, everything shifts. Children receive a steady stream of affirming messages. Over time, kids turn that respect inward. They learn to trust their bodies, feel confident in their Belonging + Identity, and approach food with the Playful Exploration that feels right to them.

Everyday Moments That Demonstrate Body Respect

- Honoring your child's hunger and fullness without pushing extra bites or limiting portions
- Welcoming your child's input on meals so they know their preferences matter
- Affirming that your child's body is good and beautiful just as it is

When Body Respect Feels Hard

Offering your child Body Respect can feel challenging if you grew up believing only certain bodies are "good" or "trustworthy." But the idea that our bodies are not inherently good and worthy is a diet culture message, designed to convince us to suppress our needs.

Remind yourself that body diversity is natural and beautiful and all bodies are wired with the capacity to care for themselves well. When we struggle, it's often because something in our environment makes true self-care harder, not because we're inherently untrustworthy. By practicing Body Respect with your child, you create a supportive space where you can both learn that all bodies are worthy, including yours.

Bringing It Home

You don't have to master every skill at once to raise a child who feels safe, seen, and confident around food. When you practice Attunement, bring a Calm and Steady Presence, and show Body Respect, you meet the needs that help your child grow into a competent, confident eater. Every time you notice their cues, steady yourself through their big feelings, and honor their body as it is, you strengthen their foundation.

For many of us, our parents didn't meet these needs, and offering what we never received can feel overwhelming. That doesn't mean you fail—it means you choose the brave work of breaking a cycle. You lead with confidence and feed with compassion when you show up with curiosity, care, and a willingness to keep trying.

The work you do matters. Even in the hardest moments, every effort you make adds up. You shape a new story for your family. By practicing these skills, you give your child the food positivity they need to thrive for life.

One Simple Step

Notice Your Struggle Spot: Next time your child has a food-related struggle, pay attention to which Guiding Skill feels most difficult for you to apply. Later, reflect on the moment and consider your next steps for strengthening this skill.

Your Food Positivity Practice
Parenting Style Check-In: *Recognizing Your Pattern*

12

Role of the Food Leader and Establishing a Food Positive Environment

I try to follow the Division of Responsibility, like dinner at six and the kitchen is closed after. But most nights my son asks for snacks before bed, and I don't know what the right move is. I spent years ignoring my own hunger, and I want my son to feel differently, but I don't know how to figure that out with these "rules" that are supposedly meant to help him have a better relationship with food than I had.

—Stefanie

IN A BOOK about feeding kids, it probably feels like we've taken a long time to get to the part about how to actually do it! But now you know why: as your child's Food Leader, you are not just responsible for what goes on their plate; you're also shaping all the supports they need to build Food Positivity.

So let's talk about *actually* feeding your kids!

The concept of a "Food Leader" is nuanced, because leadership is often confused with control. Diet culture approaches also endorse "taking charge" (read: control) over the food you serve to your kids, but the *unsupportive* strategies they recommend often look like:

- Not stocking foods in the house you don't want your kids to eat
- Avoiding certain ingredients and cooking only "clean" meals from scratch
- Teaching kids to read nutrition labels and practice portion control

And through the lens of negative values like healthism, control, and perfection, these tactics can *seem* like responsible leadership.

But that's not why you're here. You know that these tactics fuel confusion, shame, disconnection from body cues, and sometimes even eating disorders. You want something different, a way to support your child's well-being, help them eat nourishing foods, and build the Food Positivity skills they'll need to trust themselves and thrive. We do too! So let's dive into exactly how to make that happen.

The Real Work of the Food Leader

We're not going to sugarcoat it—being a truly supportive Food Leader takes *work*. Even when you're confident in your Family Core Values and Guiding Skills, the logistics of feeding well take time, attention, and care. We also know that modern life doesn't make this easy (more on that in a bit). Your responsibilities as your child's Food Leader include the following.

Providing Food

Choosing, preparing, and offering food in ways that support both nourishment and a healthy relationship with food.

Planning and Logistics *Organizing the practical side of feeding so food is reliably available without overwhelming time, energy, or resources*	• Plan, shop for, and provide meals and snacks at predictable times so your child learns food is reliable (*Attunement*). • Offer your child small, age-appropriate choices in planning (like choosing between two dinner sides) to foster confidence (*Autonomy, Developmentally Attuned*).

Safety

Creating an environment where children are physically safe and emotionally secure so they can focus on eating and connection

- Manage food allergies, choking risks, and safe food storage to keep food itself safe (*Developmentally Attuned*).
- Include at least one "safe food" your child can reliably eat at each meal so they feel anchored (*Attunement*).
- Notice your child's unique comfort needs (e.g., foods separated, softer textures, quieter setting) and adjust as you're able (*Attunement*).
- Support sleep, emotional regulation, and sensory needs so your child can come to meals ready to listen to their body (*Calm + Steady Presence, Developmentally Attuned*).

Variety and Exposure

Supporting comfort and curiosity with a wide range of foods through repeated, low-pressure opportunities

- Encourage exploration without pressure by letting your child play, smell, or touch food before tasting (*Playful Exploration*).
- Celebrate family and cultural foods to show that your child's identity belongs at the table (*Belonging + Identity, Inclusive*).
- Model your own enjoyment of a variety of foods so your child sees food as joyful and safe (*Experience-Based + Joyful*).

Nutrition

Ensuring children consistently receive enough food and nutrients to support growth, energy, and well-being

- Serve nutrient-dense foods often enough so your child can get used to feeling the benefits of being well-fueled (*Self-Regulation, Calm + Steady Presence*).
- Serve highly palatable foods regularly enough that they feel ordinary, not "special" (*Self-Regulation, Attunement, Body Respect*).
- Set thoughtful limits on foods when needed for balance or practicality, while still affirming your child's needs (*Attunement, Calm + Steady Presence*).
- Highlight how foods support energy, focus, and comfort in ways your child can understand (*Developmentally Attuned, Body Positive*).

Food Environment

Shaping mealtimes so they support eating, connection, and a sense of belonging.

Physical Setting *Ensuring that the spaces where your child eats support their physical needs*	• Create a calm and low-distraction environment in line with your child's sensory needs so they can focus on eating and connection at the table (*Attunement, Calm + Steady Presence*).
	• Ensure your child has age-appropriate, comfortable seating that supports their body so mealtime feels secure and manageable (*Developmentally Attuned*).
	• Invite your child to contribute to the setup, like placing napkins, choosing background music, or picking a centerpiece (*Autonomy*).
	• Keep kid-friendly tools like small tongs, fun utensils or colorful plates available so kids can serve themselves and explore food in hands-on ways (*Autonomy, Experience-Based + Joyful*).
Emotional Setting *Creating environments where children can eat comfortably, safely, and with positive association*	• Remove pressure, shame, or coercion from mealtimes (*Autonomy, Attunement, Calm + Steady Presence, Body Respect*).
	• Help your child feel safe and comfortable at the table, to associate food experiences with security and belonging (*Belonging + Identity, Attunement*).
	• Acknowledge and validate emotions that show up at the table, like with *"I hear that you're disappointed the food looks different today"* (*Calm + Steady Presence*).
	• Show respect for all appetites and bodies by avoiding judgment or comparison (*Body Respect, Belonging + Identity, Inclusive*).
	• Allow humor, stories, or playful conversation to create a sense of joy and safety around food (*Playful Exploration, Experience-Based + Joyful*).
	• Celebrate and name cultural and family food traditions at meals (*Belonging + Identity, Inclusive*).
	• Let your child lead a food "experiment" at the table once in a while, like mixing two foods together to see what happens (*Autonomy, Playful Exploration*).

Structure and Flexibility

Providing reliable patterns with meals and snacks, while staying responsive to real-life needs.

Structure	
Creating a reliable rhythm of meals and snacks so children feel secure that food will be offered consistently and predictably	• Provide consistent, reliable access to meals and snacks so your child learns that food is dependable (*Attunement, Calm + Steady Presence, Body Respect*).
	• Plan meal times around your child's natural hunger rhythms (like after school) so they come to the table ready to eat (*Attunement, Calm + Steady Presence*).
	• Use predictable routines (same times, family rituals) to anchor children in a sense of belonging and trust (*Belonging + Identity, Body Respect*).
	• Narrate routines in simple, age-appropriate ways, like "We'll have dinner after playtime" so kids connect timing with their body signals (*Self-Regulation, Developmentally Attuned*).
Flexibility	
Meeting children's food needs in a responsive and attuned way outside of set meal and snack times, so children learn that food is nourishing and joyful, not rigid	• Respect that appetites change day to day (growth spurts, energy levels) and adjust without shame or pressure (*Body Respect*).
	• Respond with curiosity instead of frustration when requests come outside meal times, like saying "I wonder if you're hungry or just needing a break" (*Attunement, Calm + Steady Presence*).
	• Trust your child's genuine hunger/fullness cues even when they don't match the planned schedule (*Attunement, Body Respect*).
	• Use flexibility moments as practice for independence, like letting kids prep a simple snack (*Autonomy, Developmentally Attuned*).

Respect and Guidance

Building a trusting, attuned partnership with your child that fosters their ability to eat what they need and explore food at their own pace

Connection & Trust *Encouraging your child's sense of security, autonomy, and trust in the feeding relationship*	• Allow your child to decide how much to eat from what's provided, reinforcing that their body's signals are trustworthy (*Attunement, Body Respect*). • Create predictable rituals, like a family blessing, gratitude, or check-in, so meals feel like moments of belonging (*Belonging + Identity*). • Use rituals like sharing "the funniest thing about our day" or telling food stories to make mealtimes feel joyful and safe (*Experience-Based + Joyful*).
Skill Building *Encouraging your child's development of eating skills and confidence with food*	• Provide opportunities for age-appropriate motor skill development (chewing, self-feeding, utensil use, new textures) so eating feels safe and manageable at every stage (*Developmentally Attuned*). • Offer stepwise challenges (like mixing ingredients before tasting) matched to the child's age and stage (*Developmentally Attuned*). • Encourage playful practice, like stacking crackers or sniffing spices (*Playful Exploration*). • Let children take leadership in small tasks, like choosing toppings serving their own portions (*Autonomy*). • Invite your child to share observations about their body or appetite, like saying "How does your tummy feel after that snack?" (*Self-Regulation*). • Connect food skills to family traditions, like a grandparent's recipe or holiday food prep (*Belonging + Identity*). • Treat learning to cook or serve themselves as hands-on adventures, like letting them measure, stir, or plate foods their way, even if it gets messy (*Autonomy, Experience-Based + Joyful*). • Introduce simple meal planning or cooking tasks like choosing a recipe or measuring ingredients to build lifelong confidence with food (*Autonomy, Developmentally Attuned*).

Modeling	• Eat the food you need to support your own well-being
Demonstrating	and avoid restrictive or weight-focused behaviors
through your own	(*Calm + Steady Presence, Body Respect*).
behavior what	• Show curiosity by trying new foods yourself, even
Food Positivity	imperfectly (*Playful Exploration, Experience-*
looks like	*Based + Joyful*).
	• Use respectful food and body language aloud (*Body Respect, Body Positive*).
	• Demonstrate flexibility, like saying "I'm not very hungry tonight, so I'll save this for later" (*Self-Regulation*).
	• Normalize silliness and imperfection, like laughing at your own "cooking fails" or food experiments gone wrong so food feels fun, not pressured (*Playful Exploration*).
	• Share genuine enjoyment of meals, like "This ice cream is really hitting the spot!" to model that food is about comfort and pleasure, not just nutrients (*Body Respect, Experience-Based + Joyful*).

Taking It All In

It's understandable if this list feels overwhelming. The truth is, positive Food Leadership does take significant time and energy, but these investments are what make it so powerful for your child. This is also why we place such an emphasis on the role of the SDoH. How can you realistically shop for, plan, and cook balanced meals that align with your child's unique needs, all while applying the Guiding Skills (and feeding yourself, too!) when you're exhausted, lacking support, or stretched thin financially?

If that's your reality, please hear us out: Our goal is not to put additional pressure on you. Just as kids need Felt Safety before they can grow Food Positivity, *you* also need a foundation of physical, emotional, and financial support to step into Food Leadership. If that foundation is shaky right now, we encourage you to seek the supports available to you—whether that's food assistance, more support from your co-parent, or simply showing yourself compassion when feeding just feels *hard*.

Bonus Handout via the QR Code: Co-parenting with Food Positivity

It's also worth noting that the long list of the Food Leader's responsibilities is one more reason that control-oriented and permissive feeding approaches can feel so tempting. They shrink the parent's task list. Control-oriented feeding simplifies feeding to "Here's what you can eat, deal with it," while permissive feeding pares it down to "Eat whatever and whenever."

In the moment, either approach can feel easier, especially when you're under stress. But over time, they create conflict and confusion, and they don't support your child in developing Food Positivity.

The Division of Responsibility

Looking at the Food Leader's responsibilities, you may notice that the first three categories (Providing Food, Food Environment, and Structure and Flexibility) align with the *what, when,* and *where* your child eats.

What you don't see on the list is any responsibility for *whether* your child eats a certain food you offer or, if they do choose to eat it, *how much* they need to eat to feel full. In fact, in the last category (Respect and Guidance), your responsibilities specifically include letting your child make these choices.

This sharing of feeding responsibilities between parent and child is well-known in child feeding research as Ellyn Satter's Division of Responsibility (DOR). And if you've spent any time on the internet looking for advice on how to feed your kids, you've probably already come across it.

DOR Parent Responsibilities	DOR Child Responsibilities
What, when, and *where* of food	*Whether* and *how much* to eat

Decades of research show its effectiveness in helping children to both eat well and develop a healthy relationship with food for life. When kids are given both structure and autonomy through DOR, they're more likely to eat a variety of nutrient-dense foods, regulate their intake according to hunger and fullness, and have positive experiences at mealtimes.

We strongly support DOR for managing the day-to-day side of feeding within your overall Food Positive approach. The DOR framework especially helps you to make decisions to support your child's nutrition and avoid the overwhelm of short order cooking, along with many of the other practical elements of the Food Leader's responsibilities.

DOR is also known as the "Trust Model," for reasons that align perfectly with Food Positivity. The child trusts that the parent will meet their needs and the parent trusts that the child is capable of thriving under their leadership.

> "You simply can't have it both ways. If you try to be a little bit controlling and a little bit trusting, you will end up controlling, utterly confuse yourself and make your child unhappy."
>
> —Ellyn Satter, "Secrets of Feeding a Healthy Family"

But here's the nuance: DOR works only when those two things are actually happening. Influenced by the unsupportive values and parenting tactics we grew up with, so many of us just don't have the skills to parent in a way that builds trust by truly meeting our children's underlying needs—not only at the table but in every aspect of family life. And diet culture teaches us to believe that humans truly cannot self-regulate their food intake. How can we trust our kids to do so when we've never believed it about ourselves?

The Division of Responsibility Gone Wrong

Because of the doubts and fears we struggle to let go of, DOR is often used in ways that don't actually reflect attuned leadership rooted in positive values. The pull of diet culture is strong, and many popular interpretations of DOR—especially on social media—focus on "reversing picky eating" or "getting" kids to eat, never acknowledging that neither of these are the goals Satter intended.

"Kid Food Instagram has taught us that we have to retain total control over the family meal experience because our side of the Division of Responsibility bargain matters more than our kids' role."

—Virginia Sole-Smith, "What Instagram Gets Wrong About Feeding Your Kids," Burnt Toast

And because of the ways diet culture has harmed our *own* relationships with food, we also end up using DOR as a stand-in for our own judgment. When that happens, it ends up mirroring precisely how we outsource our own decisions about what to eat to diet plans. This misuse of DOR doesn't support our children either. It reinforces the same unhelpful patterns we're trying to leave behind.

Let's take a look at some of the ways that misusing DOR does not actually support our kids:

Common Misapplication	Parent's Likely Intention	How It Violates the Child's Needs	The Nuance
Adhering rigidly to meal and snack schedule	Cut down on total food intake by eliminating eating between meals	Your child feels unsupported and learns to distrust their body cues, weakening Felt Safety and Self-Regulation.	A predictable meal schedule promotes Felt Safety, but your child also needs your Attunement to when they are truly hungry outside of those times.
Using the "what" responsibility as a loophole for restriction	Ensure that only "healthy" food is available to the child	Your child feels deprived, which can fuel preoccupation with restricted items and harms Autonomy and Belonging + Identity.	Parents should guide the child's overall nutrition, but the child's curiosity and satisfaction with food matters, too.

Common Misapplication	Parent's Likely Intention	How It Violates the Child's Needs	The Nuance
Serving foods with the objective of "getting" the kids to like them	Hoping repeated exposure will guarantee acceptance and prevent picky eating	Your child feels pressured to eat what's served and that their preferences don't matter, discouraging Playful Exploration and their sense of Belonging + Identity.	Repeated exposure does help children develop an interest in new foods, but there will still be plenty of foods they simply don't like.
Deferring to the "rules" of DOR instead of your own Attunement to your child's needs	Feeling unsure about their own instincts and hoping that outsourcing decisions to DOR will safeguard their child's relationship with food	Your child feels unseen when you don't respond to their cues, reducing their sense of Felt Safety, Body Trust and Autonomy and making eating feel more about rules than connection.	DOR is most effective when parents themselves feel comfortable and confident with food. If a parent relies heavily on external rules, it's impossible to prioritize Attunement to the child's needs.

If any of this has been your experience with DOR, once again—it's not your fault. Diet culture robbed you of the skills and understanding you needed to use the model effectively. And whether or not you've ever even heard of DOR, just by reading this book you are taking the time to learn how to *genuinely* support your child.

Food Positivity gives you these tools. And when it comes to DOR, rejecting control-oriented values through your Family Core Values and meeting your child's Growing Needs through your Attunement, Calm + Steady Presence, and Body Respect helps you build the trusting relationship with your child that allows Satter's model to work as intended.

Limits and Boundaries: Your Tools for Positive Leadership

Once we let go of control, we can finally use DOR for good. And just like every other aspect of parenting, you'll often need to make decisions your child isn't very happy about. We're not talking about the misapplications mentioned earlier, though. We're talking about the things you genuinely need to do to support your child—everything from offering balanced meals to keeping cracker crumbs out of your couch cushions.

It's tricky to tell the difference at first. A diet extremely high in sugar, for example, doesn't leave room for the other nutrients your child needs to thrive. It's okay, even necessary at times, to gently limit sugar (or any other food significantly out of balance) for your child to eat more variety and get the nutrients they need. But if your limit on sugar results in the child rarely getting to enjoy it at all, then it compromises their Felt Safety, Autonomy, and Self-Regulation.

Figuring out the right choice takes time, but with practice you'll begin to notice when your choices are rooted in genuine attunement to your child's well-being versus when they're coming from fear and control.

Even your most supportive limits will frustrate your child. And that's actually a good thing! Children are wired to push limits—it's how they figure out what's safe, what they can expect, and where they can exert their Autonomy. Pushing back isn't defiance so much as a way to test whether their caregivers are consistent and dependable. When you hold steady, it reassures the child: "My world is safe and predictable. My grown-up will take care of me."

Think of a child who is clearly tired but protests going to sleep. They don't yet have the cognitive ability to think, "I'm tired, and going to sleep now will help me have a good day tomorrow." Instead, they may show their need for sleep through crying or acting out. In that moment, you lovingly guide them to bed and move through a predictable bedtime routine, holding steady to the boundaries you've established that support their need for rest. That consistency not only helps them get the rest they need, but also gives them the security of knowing they can rely on your care until they're ⸲ to handle bedtime on their own.

We can treat food the same way. Here are some examples of limits and boundaries you might hold relating to food, keeping in mind that your Attunement to your child's individual needs always comes first:

- "Please put those chips back, I'm about to serve dinner."
- "Remember, we don't eat in the living room. Let's bring those pretzels to the table so we can eat them here together."
- "I'm saving the rest of our grapes for another meal, but there are still other foods on the table you can eat until you're full."

When your child gets frustrated, remember that's part of the process. We'll explore how to handle those conversations in Part IV.

Do Parental Boundaries Support Intuitive Eating?

Some parents worry that leaving the responsibilities of *whether* and *how much* to their child won't support them in getting the nutrition they need. Others worry that taking over the *what, when,* and *where* of a child's food is too restrictive and interferes with their natural intuitive eating ability.

The truth is, while children are born with the ability to sense hunger, fullness, and their readiness to try a new food, what they don't yet have is the maturity to meet all of their self-care needs alone. That's where you come in, guiding the *what, when, and where* of eating until they're developmentally ready to handle these responsibilities themselves.

Interestingly, the adult framework of Intuitive Eating (developed by Evelyn Tribole and Elyse Resch to help adults heal from

(continued)

(*continued*)

chronic dieting) actually reinforces this concept. Adults learning Intuitive Eating generally experiment with a "free for all" style of eating early in the process, only to discover that structures like regular mealtimes and choosing foods that provide energy for the day ahead actually make eating feel *better*. They choose to implement boundaries with *themselves* as an act of their own self-care.

In the same way, supportive structures in childhood aren't a violation of your child's natural abilities, they're the training ground. With your guidance, kids get to practice their Growing Skills in an environment of safety and trust, so they'll never even need the Intuitive Eating framework as adults.

And while your boundaries are the part of DOR that will most test your child, trusting them with the "whether" and "how much" will almost certainly be the part that will most test *you*.

But think about it this way: your child's responsibilities are their boundaries with *you*, the way they keep *themselves* safe. This can feel deeply uncomfortable, especially if practicing Body Respect is new to you or something you've struggled to extend to yourself. But by honoring those boundaries, you strengthen your child's Body Trust and open the door to Food Positivity.

Beyond DOR: Centering the Whole-Child

There are a few ways Food Positivity goes a bit further than DOR, however. With the ultimate goals of responsive parenting in mind—things like secure attachment, emotional regulation, and respecting your child as a valued member of your family—we encourage using DOR in a reciprocal way that is attuned to your unique child.

So while DOR generally encourages family meals, we know that some children will do better eating with a screen or without the stimulation of other family members eating nearby. Another piece of DOR is offering variety and serving the parent's preferred foods often, but we know that a child with ARFID or who has experienced trauma may indeed need you to serve *their* limited, preferred foods often enough that they can eat what they need.

In every case, you're still taking responsibility for exactly what, when, and where to feed your child, but you are doing so through Attunement to the child in front of you, in a way that meets their unique Growing Needs.

You don't have to accommodate your child's every last desire, of course. Some requests won't be practical, and saying no to others provides the challenges you know your child is ready for that we explored in the previous chapter. What's most important is using your Attunement to understand what your child is communicating to you about their food needs and interests, even if they never say it out loud. You may consider, "Does my child need more opportunities to enjoy sweets in unlimited amounts?" or "Perhaps I should buy extra grapes on my next grocery run."

And as your child grows and becomes more able to share their food interests, Food Positivity encourages you to go above and *beyond* DOR in the ways you support your child's Growing Skills. That could look like the following:

> *When you meet your child's Growing Needs, you build the trust DOR depends on. And when you support their Guiding Needs, you go even further, into the full practice of Food Positivity.*

Growing Skill	Examples
Autonomy	Adding their favorite meals into your dinner rotation so they know "their pick" is on the menu.
	Offering choices, like asking if they'd like pasta with pesto or marinara, so they can practice making food decisions.
Self-Regulation	Checking in on snack timing, like asking if they feel ready now or would like to wait until after finishing a game or activity.
	Encouraging them to notice how food feels in their body, like asking, "Do you feel more energized after that sandwich or the fruit?" so they can practice connecting their appetite with their body signals.

(continued)

(*continued*)

Growing Skill	Examples
Playful Exploration	Buying a snack their friend had at school so they can see how it stacks up against their other favorites.
	Letting them suggest silly food experiments, like seeing what happens when you put popcorn in soup or dipping fruit in salsa.
Belonging + Identity	Tweaking meal prep for them, like a "build-your-own" version of your meal with the parts separate to match their preferences.
	Bringing in foods connected to their world, like something they read about in a book or saw on a show.

Doing these things shows your child that they are a respected member of your family, with a voice that matters and a body that can be trusted. When you weave the Growing Skills into your family's food culture—by honoring your child's preferences, encouraging their curiosity, and celebrating their individuality—you send the message that *their* needs matter and that food can be a source of joy, connection, and belonging for everyone.

Connection at the Table—and Everywhere Else

You've probably heard that regular family meals are one of the best things you can do for your kids. And it's true: DOR encourages family meals because research shows that kids who share family meals tend to eat a wider variety of foods, develop strong social and emotional skills, and even have a lower risk of disordered eating down the road.

But let's be honest—family meals can also feel like one more impossible expectation. Cooking every night? Managing different food preferences? Juggling homework, sports, and bedtime? That's a *lot*. And you're not failing if regular family meals aren't your reality.

The thing is, family meals aren't just about food and a table. They matter because they're an opportunity to practice the 3 Ms and shape your child's Invisible Curriculum. But meals certainly aren't the only time you're able to strengthen your child's Food Positivity Protective Shield.

Family meals "work" only if they actually work for *you*. They're valuable because they're an opportunity to connect with your child—not because they check some cultural box of what a "good parent" does.

Bringing It Home

At this point, it's clear that feeding is about much more than what's on your child's plate. Being your child's Food Leader is no small task. It means juggling logistics, planning meals, holding boundaries, *and* modeling Food Positivity yourself, all while staying attuned to your child's needs and often working through your own. It's a lot. And it's even harder when you don't have the support and resources every family deserves.

Every time you show up as the predictable Food Leader, you're modeling something bigger than what's on the table. Food Positivity is here to help; it lays the foundation that allows DOR to work, while also giving you ways to honor your child's individuality, curiosity, and sense of belonging that will support their trust in food and their body as they grow.

One Simple Step

Think of one food-related limit or boundary that feels hard for you to hold. Pause and notice what makes you feel unsure. Is it concern over upsetting your child? Worries that your limits might be stemming from diet culture rather than your child's needs? Reflect on the reason behind the boundary and whether it truly supports your child.

Your Food Positivity Practice

Everyday Leadership: *Habits That Build Trust Kids Can Feel*

13

When Feeding Is Difficult: Supporting the Child in Front of You

It feels like all my son thinks about is food. The moment he wakes up, he's asking what he can eat. He sneaks it into his room. The more I try to rein things in, the more fixated he gets. But I can't just let him eat as much as he wants, can I? I want to help him, but I feel like I've made food into an obsession.

—Monica

YOU NOW HAVE a sense of what it means to parent—and feed—from a place of connection, structure, and trust. But even when we know *what* to do, the *how* can feel incredibly hard. Feeding kids three to five times a day, seven days a week, 365 days a year is a lot for anyone. And while it's one thing to understand the big-picture needs of children, when we add in mealtime challenges, it's quite another to stay focused on the unique needs of *your* child. Parents often share the same questions with us (and chances are, they're the ones you're asking too):

- *Am I messing this up?*
- *What if my child's eating never changes?*
- *How does this work when my child has unique needs?*

The truth is, there's no such thing as a "typical" eater. Every child brings their own preferences, challenges, and sometimes medical needs to the table. What works for one child might have the opposite effect for another. Feeding differences—whether rooted in personality, past experiences, sensory sensitivities, or health conditions—can make even the most well-meaning advice feel impossible to apply. This chapter is here to hold space for that reality.

The Food Positivity Framework guides you through the messier, more complex parts of feeding. It supports you in honoring *your* child's individuality while still raising them to trust their body, enjoy food, and grow into a confident eater.

Special Note: While this chapter offers tools and encouragement, it's not a substitute for individualized care. If your family is navigating a medical condition or a feeding difference that feels too big to manage alone, you deserve support from a complete feeding team. That includes a pediatrician, dietitian, psychologist, speech-language pathologist (SLP), and occupational therapist (OT).

The Long Game of Feeding

When feeding is difficult, it's easy to get caught up in the short term: *just one more bite, just make it through this meal, just get the veggies in, you've already had enough carbs.* But kids are always learning, whether or not they eat what we want them to eat.

It makes sense that when your child is facing a scary challenge like celiac disease, diabetes, or ARFID, you are incredibly worried for their well-being. Those fears stem from how deeply you love your child, not diet culture. But all the same, while restriction, pressure, or shaming may change their eating habits today, these tactics don't build trust for tomorrow.

You are nurturing your child now the way they will learn to nurture *themselves* as adults. What we do in these hard moments—the complex, complicated parts of feeding—is what teaches our kids the self-care skills they need to one day manage their unique needs on their own. We're equipping them with skills that last a lifetime: to nourish themselves physically, emotionally, and socially. This is Food Positivity—the long game.

Shifting from Control to Exploration

Diet culture tells parents their job is to "get" kids to eat certain foods, in certain amounts, at certain times. That message creates anxiety, and anxious feeding almost always leads to more resistance.

Food Positivity invites a shift: from control to exploration. Instead of asking, "How do I make my child eat what they're supposed to?" we ask, "How do I create an environment where my child feels safe enough to explore food and learn what they truly need?"

That one shift changes everything. Your child doesn't need to be forced, bribed, or shamed. They need support, structure, and freedom to learn at their own pace, in their own way.

Universal Supports: What Helps Every Child

Even though every child is unique, there are certain supports that help across the board. In Chapter 9 we introduced the Food Positivity Learning Foundations: Developmentally Attuned, Experience-Based and Joyful, Body Positive, and Inclusive. The following sections highlight how those same foundations apply to feeding differences.

Developmentally Attuned: Meet Them Where They Are (DA)

Feeding and learning about food look different at every stage. Babies rely on milk. Toddlers say "no" on repeat. Older kids crave independence. When we line up our expectations with where our child actually is, not where we wish they were, food feels safe, doable, and meaningful. Every phase, whether it's a picky streak or a big developmental leap, is part of how they grow.

Body Positive: Teaching Without Shame (BP)

Kids learn best about food and bodies when the lessons spark curiosity, instead of criticism. Appetites may vary, preferences will shift, and everyBODY is unique and grows on its own timeline. By respecting body cues and celebrating differences, kids get the message: *My body is good. I can trust it.* That's how Body Positivity turns everyday food moments into confidence and connection.

Experience-Based + Joyful: Play Is the Learning (E-B+J)

Kids don't learn about food by sitting still and listening. They learn when they stir, squish, sniff, and laugh. Even poking at a food or treating a real potato like Mr. Potato and playing pretend, counts as real learning. The goal isn't to "get" a bite in; it's to create playful, low-pressure moments that make food feel safe, fun, and worth exploring. That's what builds comfort and confidence over time.

Inclusive: Belonging Exactly as They Are (I)

Every child deserves to feel like they belong at the table by being welcomed to show up fully as themselves. For one child, that might mean a safe food always on the plate. For another, it's seeing their cultural dish celebrated instead of judged. When kids know their food, body, and traditions are valued, they learn the powerful truth: *Who I am belongs here.*

Regular Meals and Snacks: A Constant Across Feeding Differences

Children thrive when they can count on predictable meals and snacks. That doesn't always mean sitting at the table with you every time, but it does mean knowing that food will be offered regularly by a trusted adult. For most kids, open access to food or grazing doesn't support Self-Regulation. There are exceptions, like a child with Pathological Demand Avoidance (PDA) or past food insecurity, but consistency and rhythm are protective for the majority.

Being consistently well-nourished is also the first step to managing any feeding challenge. When kids face these situations undernourished, their bodies and brains slip into dysregulation, and frustration takes the wheel. Predictable meals and snacks give kids the fuel and stability they need so that trying a new food or sitting through a family meal feels manageable, not overwhelming.

__Bonus Handout via the QR Code:__ Diet Culture Traps That Don't Help

When Your Voice Becomes Their Voice

One of the most powerful things to remember is that the way you talk about food and their body becomes your child's inner voice. If they grow up hearing "you're picky" or "you can't control yourself," it becomes the story they believe about themselves.

And when kids believe those labels, they may start acting in ways that match them. A child called "picky" may avoid new foods, not because they *can't* try them but because they've come to believe that's just who they are. Over time, these labels shape how kids see themselves and what they believe they're capable of.

But the opposite is also true. When kids hear messages like "You're curious" or "You're still learning" or "Your body knows what it needs," they can grow into *those* identities instead.

The words you use today become their self-talk tomorrow. That's part of building their Protective Shield, the inner filter that helps them question outside messages and stay grounded in Body Trust.

From "Picky" to Learning Eater

Most parents use the word *picky* without thinking twice. But the thing is, there isn't a clear, universally accepted definition for "picky eating," "fussy eating," or "selective eating." In general, it's described as eating a limited variety of foods and refusing many others, both new and familiar.

Diet culture tells us that "good eaters" should clean their plates (but not eat too much, of course) and that if kids don't, parents must "fix" it. But a child might be cautious about food for many reasons. It's often a normal part of development, not defiance. It's how kids discover their taste bud and texture preferences and how they protect themselves when the world feels overwhelming.

Calling a child "picky" doesn't explain *why* they're cautious around certain foods. It doesn't help us understand what they need or how to support themselves. All it really does is leave both kids and parents feeling stuck.

For this reason, we don't believe in the concept or the label of "picky eating." We need language that shifts the focus. Instead of seeing feeding struggles as a fixed trait or kids as "good" versus "bad" eaters, we can choose to see eating as a process of exploring, practicing, and learning.

That's why we call kids *Learning Eaters* instead. Just like kids don't play an instrument perfectly on day one, they don't instantly accept every food. Every time they see, smell, or play with a food, they're building new skills. And when we frame it as learning, it keeps the door open for change and growth.

> Knowing why your child avoids certain foods changes the way you respond. It's not about "fixing" them. It's about meeting them where they are.

Four Common Types of Learning Eaters

Every Learning eater is different, but here are a few patterns you might recognize:

1. **Personal preference:** Just like adults, some kids have strong likes and dislikes. These preferences tend to stay the same, instead of fading or improving as kids grow, and isn't a sign of deeper issues.
2. **Sensory differences:** Certain textures, smells, or temperatures may feel overwhelming. This is common for neurodivergent kids but can show up in any child.
3. **Autonomy-seekers:** Saying "no" to food may be less about the food itself and more about practicing independence. Kids who feel pressured—whether at the table or beyond—often push

back when it comes to what they eat to protect their sense of control.

4. **Past negative experience:** A memory of choking, gagging, or being pressured can make a child fearful. This kind of avoidance is a coping strategy, not misbehavior.

When Chewing or Swallowing Is the Hard Part

If your child pockets food in their cheek, tires easily while chewing, avoids mixed textures, or gags on small lumps, the issue may not be "picky eating." It could be an oral-motor challenge. A speech-language pathologist (SLP) or occupational therapist (OT) trained in feeding can assess chewing, tongue movement, and swallowing safety.

Try saying: *"We'll keep foods easy to manage while we practice skills."*

Will They Get Enough Nutrients?

This is one of the biggest fears parents carry. Here's some reassurance: research consistently shows that most learning eaters still grow well and don't develop serious nutrient deficiencies. Kids generally find ways to meet their needs within the foods they do eat.

That said, as the Food Leader, it's important to keep an eye on their eating patterns. Many kids prefer snack-type foods because they are predictable in taste and texture. It's also common for kids to avoid whole food groups like meat, beans, eggs, produce, and/or dairy. Over time, a limited variety of foods can leave gaps in meeting their nutrient needs.

Food Neophobia: The Fear of New Foods

Many kids go through a stage of food neophobia (fear of new foods), especially in toddlerhood. Think of it like learning to swim; most kids don't dive straight into the deep end. They start with looking, smelling, or touching food long before tasting. Curiosity counts just as much as eating.

Food Positivity in Action: Learning Eaters

- Match your mealtime support to the level of stress. If mealtimes feel tense, stick mostly to preferred foods. Then slowly add new foods to explore when you think they are ready. (DA)
- Spark curiosity with exploration and playful experiences outside the table. Try visiting a farmers market, getting your hands dirty in the garden, or even placing googly eyes on a new-to-them veggie and leave it out on the counter. (E-B+J)
- Model what you experience with different tastes and textures, then ask them: "What did it taste like to you?" (BP)
- Invite their input by having them help plan meals or pick a veggie for the grocery list. (I)

Real-Life Example

Imagine you serve pasta with sauce, broccoli, and your child's favorite crackers. Your child refuses everything except the crackers.

- **Old script (pressure):** "You need to take at least one bite of broccoli before you get more crackers."
- **Food Positivity script:** Serve dinner. "How was your day?" "Oh, I just picked up some grapes; should I rinse those and put them on the table?"

If they stick with crackers? That's okay. Saying less can make a huge difference to reduce pressure at the table and over time, with repeated pressure-free (and watching you enjoy the broccoli!) helps it feel less intimidating.

Low Appetite: When They Just Don't Eat Much

Learning eating sometimes overlaps with low appetite, but some kids simply don't seem that hungry. They might skip meals, nibble tiny portions, or push food away quickly. A skipped meal once in a while is normal. But when low intake happens consistently, it can raise real concerns about your child's growth. Low appetite can be linked to temperament, medical issues, anxiety, sensory sensitivities, or even ADHD medications that suppress hunger.

When Is It More Than Learning Eating?

For many kids, being a learning eater is a normal part of development. But in some cases, the pattern may point to a deeper issue like Avoidant/Restrictive Food Intake Disorder (ARFID) or Pediatric Feeding Disorder (PFD).

ARFID is a clinical eating disorder characterized by restrictive eating that leads to nutritional, physical, or psychosocial challenges but is not driven by body image concerns. PFD is a broader medical diagnosis describing feeding issues with nutritional, developmental, sensory, or medical roots.

So how can you tell whether it's learning, eating, or something more? Here are some signs that your child's eating struggles may not be typical selective eating:

- Eating difficulties that interfere with growth, nutrition, or daily functioning
- Extremely limited accepted foods (often fewer than 20) that don't expand over time
- High anxiety around eating, even with familiar or previously liked foods
- Avoidance driven by fear (e.g., choking, vomiting, texture issues)
- Ongoing feeding struggles that create significant family stress

If you notice these patterns, reach out to a pediatrician, feeding therapist, or dietitian trained in responsive, weight-inclusive care. Getting the right support early can make a big difference—not just in nutrition but in reducing stress and rebuilding a trusting feeding relationship.

Food Positivity in Action: Low Appetite

- Speak with your pediatrician if you're worried. Many kids eat less than we expect but still grow well. (DA)
- Time big meals to when they are most hungry, such as after school or when their medication wears off. When their appetite is low, offer easy-to-eat, preferred foods. (DA)
- Tiny portions can feel less overwhelming and more inviting than large plates. (E-B+J)
- Skip the pressure. Don't bribe or say, "Just one more bite." Instead, say, "I'll help you give your body the energy it needs to run and play. Let's see what feels good today." (BP)
- Meet them where they're comfortable. If sitting at the table feels stressful, try a cozy corner or their favorite chair for meals. (I)

Real-Life Example: Low Appetite at Lunch

Your child comes home from school with a barely touched lunchbox.

- **Old script (frustrated):** "Why didn't you eat your lunch again?!? You need to eat at school."
- **Food Positivity script:** "Looks like you didn't eat much today. Let's make sure you get a snack now to help your body catch up."

This response reduces shame while still meeting the body's needs.

Body Cues, Attention, and Everything In Between

Not all feeding challenges show up as food refusals. Some kids want to eat constantly, while others are so busy they forget they need to eat. Some don't notice when they're full, and others wander into the kitchen every time they're bored. Each of these patterns can leave parents wondering: *Is this okay? Am I setting my child up for problems later?* Let's look at how to support kids whose eating looks very different from the "just right" middle ground diet culture tells us to expect.

Distracted Eaters

If you have a kiddo who "just can't sit still" or never seems to be able to stay present at the table from start to finish, you have likely experienced a distracted eater. Some kids find it almost impossible or even painful to sit at the table and stay focused on eating. Distracted eaters may fidget, jump up, or completely zone out when eating because for them, the world is far too interesting to focus just on a meal. This difference is especially common for kids with ADHD, who may already struggle with noticing when they're hungry and whose brains are wired for stimulation and movement.

Food Positivity in Action: Distracted Eaters

- Use gentle cues to transition like a timer, short song, or hand-washing ritual to signal: "Now it's time to eat." (DA)
- Keep mealtime engaging with conversation starters or a simple family game to help hold their attention without pressuring. (E-B+J)
- Invite movement as part of the meal if it helps them stay regulated. You might allow standing; an exercise ball as a seat; pre-, middle-, or post-meal dance parties; or even a fidget toy if it helps them stay calm and present. (BP)
- Normalize their supports instead of comparing them to siblings who may not need the same tools. You might say, "Timers help you stay focused and remember to eat." (I)

To Screen or Not to Screen

For some, a screen can be a supportive tool, but often it may be a sign of underlying feeding or regulation struggles. Screens may be a short-term bridge, but if they become the only strategy for mealtimes, it's worth checking in with a supportive provider.

Enthusiastic Eaters

Diet culture sends the message that we should fear and control big appetites, which leads parents to feel uneasy when their child's hunger doesn't stay within what they believe to be "normal." When a child enjoys food, eats large portions, or asks for snacks all day long, many worry their child has "no stopping point" or that they're on track for unwanted weight gain. But the truth is, appetites vary from child to child and change during periods of growth.

Few kids eat in that idealized "middle zone" of not too picky but not overly enthusiastic either, because it's a diet culture fantasy. Families may also experience conflict when one child eats more than others. A child who moves quickly through the week's snacks or wants more than their share at dinner can create tension and feelings of unfairness within the family. And just like learning eaters, this leaves the enthusiastic eater feeling that their appetite and food preferences are "wrong."

Food Positivity in Action: Enthusiastic Eaters

- Set caring limits, not fearful ones. It's okay to limit access to a single food when necessary and find a balance with offering plenty of satisfying alternatives. (DA)
- Plan for abundance by offering generous servings of favorite foods, such as unlimited cookies at snack time, to reduce scarcity and build trust. (E-B+J)
- Respect appetite differences by saying things like, "Your body knows what it needs." (BP).
- Celebrate their love of food by including them in planning family meals, treating their enthusiasm as a strength, instead of a flaw. (I)

A bigger appetite doesn't mean your child is destined for problems. Honoring their hunger teaches them to trust their body instead of fearing it.

When Kids Don't Notice Fullness

For many parents, one of the most unsettling parts of feeding is when a child doesn't seem to notice when they've had enough. Instead of stopping naturally, they may keep eating until they feel uncomfortable, leaving parents to wonder: *How can I trust my child to listen to their body if they don't seem to know when to stop?* This worry is especially heightened in a culture that treats large appetites and big bodies with suspicion. Neurodivergence, anxiety, or past restrictions can make a child's awareness of when to stop harder, too. But just like with any other feeding difference, the goal isn't to *reduce* your child's intake; it's to help them get the *right* amount of food to grow and thrive. Instead of trying to control how much they eat, shift toward helping them *tune in.*

Food Positivity in Action: When Kids Don't Notice Fullness

- Undereating early in the day often triggers overeating later in the day. By frontloading nourishment, such as offering a satisfying breakfast and snacks earlier in the day, it can help reduce overeating later. (DA)
- Pause gently with body check-ins like "Let's sip water and see how your tummy feels." They can always keep eating. (E-B+J)
- Lead with modeling by sharing when you've eaten more than you needed: "I was so full after that meal; the next time I am going to do a better job of tuning-in to my body." (BP)
- Affirm body differences by reminding them: "Everyone's fullness cues look different. You'll keep learning what yours feel like." (I)

Interoception Challenges

Some kids struggle with understanding the signals their body is sending like hunger, fullness, and even needing to use the toilet. Taking the lead with simple "body check-in" can help, especially paired with visuals. Modeling how you connect your body signals is helpful too—"My stomach is hurting, and I am feeling grouchy, I think I might be hungry." Or before a meal try: "Do you feel dizzy or have trouble focusing?" After: "Same or different now?" Visual scales (like traffic lights or smiley faces) can help kids who aren't verbal yet too.

When Kids Don't Notice Hunger

Some children may not feel hunger in typical ways, like a growling stomach. This can be especially concerning because we want to be able to trust our children's hunger cues—but what if those cues don't seem to be there? Appetite can be dulled by medication, distraction, anxiety, neurodivergence, or even past trauma that conditions kids not to notice their hunger. Getting to the root of why a child struggles with hunger awareness is important, as is noticing our child's more subtle cues signaling their need for food and helping them learn to do the same.

Beyond a Growling Stomach: Other Signs of Hunger

As adults, we often think of hunger in black-and-white terms— your stomach growls, so it must be time to eat! But children don't always experience or recognize hunger in this way. Some kids rarely notice their stomach growling at all, while others may feel it but not connect the sensation to needing to eat. Other cues signaling a child may be hungry include the following:

- Irritability or sudden mood swings
- Zoning out or trouble focusing
- Feeling tired or sluggish
- Headaches or stomach pains
- Becoming clumsy or restless

We can support our kids by noticing these cues ourselves and planning meals and snacks for these times. As they grow, we can support them in naming and noticing these same connections so they can one day recognize and respond to these cues on their own.

Food Positivity in Action: When Kids Don't Notice Hunger

- Help them learn to spot their subtle cues that they need to eat like anger, frustration, fatigue, or zoning out. (DA)
- Practice curiosity and checking in; ask: "How does your body feel right now?" before and after eating to build awareness. It also

helps to talk through your own cues, like "I'm feeling sleepy; I think I need to eat something." (E-B+J)

- Validate their experience that not everyone feels hunger in the same way and their signals are just as real. (I)
- Normalize the need for tools to support them in learning their body cues and encourage them to brainstorm things that they think would be supportive for their own body. (BP)

Eating Out of Boredom

For some kids, food becomes the go-to when they don't know what else to do. They wander into the kitchen between meals, ask for snacks right after eating, or graze whenever they have the opportunity. The parent's challenge is determining through Attunement whether the child genuinely needs more to eat or if they need additional coping skills for their boredom. This pattern is especially common for children with ADHD, who use food as a reliable source of stimulation but can show up in any child when other outlets for their energy, curiosity, or need for connection aren't available. Keep in mind that eating when bored isn't necessarily something we want to teach our kids to avoid at all costs, but they deserve to build other strategies to combat boredom as well.

Food Positivity in Action: Eating Out of Boredom

- Spot patterns. Notice when boredom hunger shows up even when they're just had a filling meal (like after school) and plan alternatives in advance. (DA)
- Notice when boredom eating might be a cry for connection with *you*, and plan time together as you are able. (DA)
- Build self-awareness by asking: "How did your body feel after snacking when you weren't hungry?" (E-B+J)
- Find activities like crafts, games, or outdoor play that can meet the same need for stimulation and connection. (BP)
- Normalize eating when you're bored by saying: "Everyone eats when they're bored sometimes. You're human. Let's find other fun things, too." (I)

Feeding Through Trauma and Sensory Overload

Some of the toughest feeding differences don't come from appetite or personality; they come from life experiences, nervous system wiring, or the way a child processes the world through their senses. These can be draining for parents, especially when every meal feels like walking on eggshells. But with the right supports, kids can rebuild safety and learn to trust both food and their bodies.

> "Yes, feeding challenges make it more difficult for children to eat, but extreme reactions to foods are often the result of anxiety, pressure, previous painful experiences, and forcing, not the fact that a bowl of applesauce is on the table."
>
> —Katja Rowell, *Love Me, Feed Me*

Trauma, Stress, and Food Insecurity

Some children's eating struggles are rooted in past or ongoing trauma, difficult life events such as a death or divorce, or a history of food insecurity or neglectful feeding. Pressuring or restrictive feeding tactics can contribute to this feeding difference as well. What looks like overeating, sneaking food, or refusing to eat is often a child's way of coping with circumstances that don't meet their basic needs. When parents or providers try to "fix" the eating behavior without addressing those underlying experiences, the struggles usually intensify. The real challenge is supporting children in rebuilding trust in food, their own bodies, and the safety of the eating experience.

Food Positivity in Action: Trauma, Stress, and Food Insecurity

- Build felt safety beyond food. Connection and a calm presence matter just as much as what's on the plate. (DA)
- Keep food exploration gentle and fun. Make meals feel steady and pressure-free so curiosity grows. (E-B+J)
- Validate stress-driven eating: "Food helps you feel safe right now, and that's okay." (BP)
- Acknowledge bigger forces by talking openly about food insecurity in developmentally attuned ways. (I)

> What looks like defiance is often fear. Your calm, consistent care can be healing.

Thriving on Predictability and Routine

Some children feel most secure when their feeding follows a steady, predictable rhythm. Familiar foods, repeated meal patterns, and consistent settings provide a sense of safety that helps them feel grounded enough to eat. While at times any child might lean on sameness when the world feels overwhelming, for many autistic children in particular, predictability is not simply a preference but a vital support for their regulation and well-being.

For parents, this can bring both reassurance and questions. It may be hard not to worry about what honoring the child's routines or their food preferences means for variety or flexibility down the road. The key is remembering that predictability is a legitimate need, not a problem to solve.

Food Positivity in Action: Thriving on Predictability and Routine

- Serve preferred foods at predictable times to reduce stress and help their body tune in. (DA)
- Introduce new foods gradually and start small. Try exploring foods with four or five senses, which can be a fun pressure-free activity. (E-B+J)
- Validating and respecting their preferences by offering repeated meals. These are valid body signals, not misbehavior. (BP)
- Include their accepted foods at family gatherings so they feel welcome and safe at the table. (I)

Sensory Needs

Some children experience the world through their senses in ways that are either more intense or less noticeable than others. For kids with sensory needs, sights, sounds, smells, textures, and movement can feel overwhelming or, in some cases, not stimulating enough.

While sensory avoiders react strongly to overwhelming textures, tastes, or noises, sensory seekers crave extra input and may use food for stimulation. Other children may be highly sensitive, noticing every small change, or under-responsive and find sensory cues that are hardly noticeable at all.

At mealtimes, sensory differences can show up as avoiding certain textures, seeking out strong flavors or crunch or being seemingly unaware of the body's signals at all. In fact, many feeding struggles may stem from sensory differences that haven't yet been identified. And while unique sensory needs are common with autism, they're not exclusive to it.

Food Positivity in Action: Sensory Needs

- Consider an evaluation by an affirming feeding therapist (OT or SLP) if you suspect your child needs support in developing skills to improve their eating. (DA)
- Offer exploration only when ready by following their lead— touching or smelling is enough until they choose to taste. (E-B+J)
- Validate sensory responses by repeating what they experience. That may sound like: "That texture feels rough to you," because their experiences are real signals. (BP)
- Prioritize inclusion by adapting family meals so their safe foods are present, and shape the environment to help them feel they belong. (I)

Bonus Handout via the QR Code: Medical Needs and Special Nutrition

Bringing It Home

While this chapter explores many common feeding differences children may experience, it's not a comprehensive guide. Every child's needs are unique and often complex or constantly changing, which is why ongoing collaboration with supportive healthcare providers can be so valuable. We'll explore this kind of collaboration in Chapter 21.

Feeding differences are part of raising a one-of-a-kind child. When you respond with true support and compassion, you're doing far more than feeding your child at the moment. You're teaching them how to care for themselves with that level of care, both now and as they grow into adulthood.

We also want to acknowledge how demanding this can be. Supporting a child with feeding differences takes time, patience, creativity, and mental and emotional energy. If you feel stretched thin, you're not alone. The fact that you continue to show up matters deeply. And remember: you deserve support, rest, and satisfying food, too.

One Simple Step

Take one moment to reframe your child's feeding difference as a part of their individuality, not a flaw. Instead of asking "How do I fix this?" use your Attunement skills. Try asking, "What is this showing me about who my child is and what they need right now?"

Your Food Positivity Practice
Feeding Differences: *Small Shifts Toward Trust*

14

Putting It All Together: The Heart of Food Positivity

It's Tuesday night. Dinner is running late, your oldest is melting down because they're "starving," and your youngest looks at the plate and says, "I don't want this."

The old script bubbles up in your head: "Too bad, this is what's for dinner." But tonight you take a breath. You remember that feeling safe matters more than winning a battle. So you slide the bread basket closer and say, "That's okay, you can start with this. Do you want to go grab the Nutella?"

Your child's shoulders soften. A few minutes later, they reach for a spoonful of rice on their own. Nothing magical, no perfectly balanced plate, just a calm moment where trust grew instead of tension.

YOU'VE JUST WORKED your way through some of the hardest truths about what it really means to feed your child well. You've thought about your family's values, your role in supporting your child's relationship with food, and the many ways eating might look different for your unique kid.

And it's a lot.

But you're already doing what matters most: You're showing up and supporting your child with care.

At its core, Food Positivity is simple: It's an approach for you and a life skill for your child.

It's the choice to make food a source of safety, trust, connection, and joy. It's the belief that your child's well-being isn't measured by what they eat at one meal but by how they feel in their body and around the table over time.

This is why we wrote this book. Every page until now has been building to this moment. You've learned where our struggles with food came from, what your child really needs, and how your presence can make all the difference. Now, here in the heart of Food Positivity, it all comes together.

Your Foundations: A Bird's-Eye View

Food Positivity is built on the four foundations that shape the way kids learn about food and their bodies: **Feeding, Parenting, Learning, and Environment**.

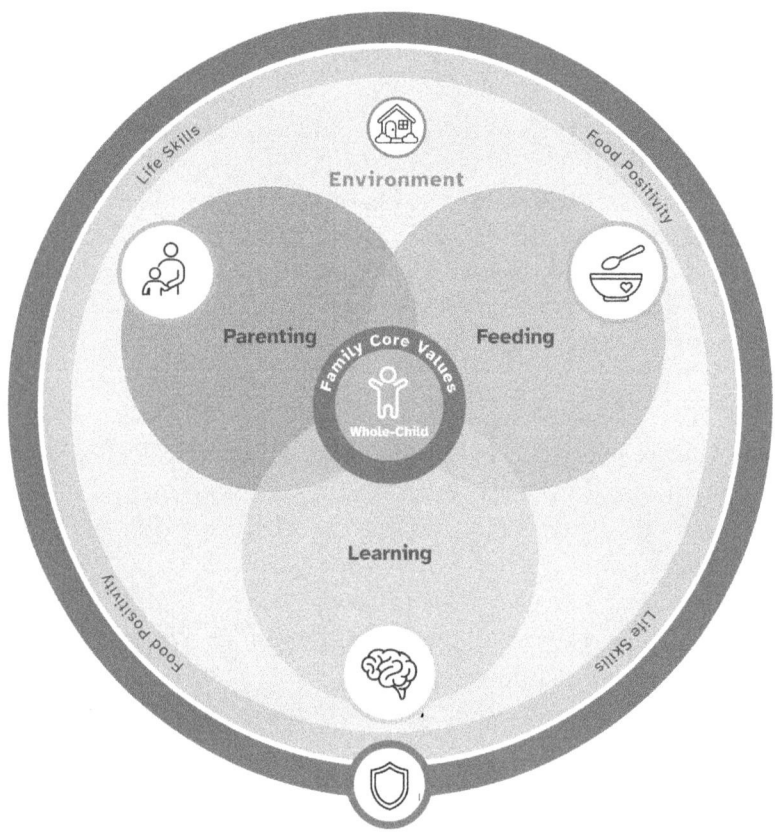

Think of these as the key areas of family life. They overlap and blend together, because life with kids is a "messy intersection." Feeding is never *just* feeding; it's also parenting, because *how* you show up matters. It's also learning, because every meal is a lesson in disguise. And all of it unfolds inside an environment that never turns off.

Here's what each foundation means in real life:

- **Feeding** is about how kids experience food. Not just *what's* on the plate, but *how* it's offered. Is there pressure, or is there safety? Is there shame, or is there curiosity? Feeding moments are the stage where trust (or fear) takes root.
- **Parenting** is about how you guide and connect with your child. Every tone of voice, every response to a meltdown, every choice to stay calm or pile on pressure—all of it teaches your child something about themselves and about food.
- **Learning** is how kids actually grow skills. Children don't learn about food from charts or lectures; they learn by exploring, playing, repeating, and reflecting. Every sensory experience, every sticky kitchen experiment, every "just watching for now" is part of the learning process.
- **Environment** is the backdrop always teaching. The words you use about your own body, the routines that make food feel predictable, the quiet tone at the table. . .these are the invisible lessons. We lovingly call this Invisible Curriculum the 3 Ms (Modeling, Messaging, and Moments), and that's because whether you notice it or not, they're always in the background shaping what your child absorbs.

When you put all four foundations together, you start to see the bigger picture: Your child isn't just learning about food or bodies in one place or one way. They're learning in every bite, every conversation, every choice, and every moment.

Your Framework: Close-Up View

The four foundations hold the Food Positivity Framework together, but as you read through each of the foundations in Part II and Part III, you may have been wondering: *What's actually happening inside those foundations? How does all of this play out for me and my child at the table, in the kitchen, or on a busy Tuesday night?*

This is where the overall Food Positivity Framework comes in. It's the map showing you how to move through everyday moments with more clarity and confidence.

At the center is your child—the Whole-Child, with their unique needs, strengths, and sensitivities. Wrapped around them are your Family Core Values, the compass that helps you find your way when decisions feel hard. From there, the layers move outward into your child's needs and skills, the guidance you bring, and the environment that surrounds it all. Over time, those everyday layers build toward something powerful: a protective shield your child carries with them into the world.

The Whole-Child

At the center is your child's whole self, not just their appetite or what they eat at dinner but their personality, preferences, interests, and feelings.

When we see feeding through this lens, dinner isn't just about salad or bread; it's also about connection, curiosity, and belonging. It's about respecting who your child is today while helping them grow into who they're becoming.

That's why every part of the framework wraps around the Whole-Child. When kids feel safe, valued, and understood, they're able to explore food and their bodies with confidence.

Family Core Values: Your Compass

Your Family Core Values are the things you care about most, the beliefs that guide how you parent, and the tone you set at the table.

Getting clear on your values is like holding a compass. When decisions around food and bodies feel tricky, like dessert before dinner, comments from grandparents, or a child declaring, "I'm fat," your values help shape the way you respond without second-guessing.

Your values might be about respect, kindness, curiosity, inclusion, faith, or connection. Whatever they are, they "hug" your child, shaping the way you respond in everyday moments. And over time, they become the compass your child learns to carry for themselves, a tool they'll use to navigate food and body messages for the rest of their life.

Growing Needs ↔ Guiding Needs

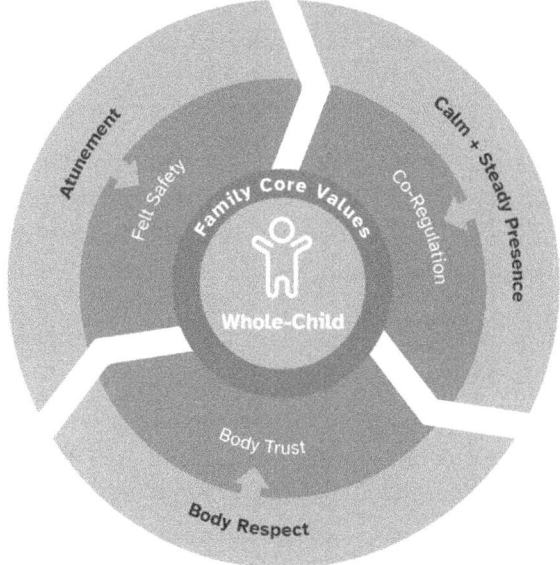

The next layer is about Needs: your child's Growing Needs and your Guiding Needs as the parent.

Kids have certain emotional Growing Needs that have to be met before they can truly learn, explore, or build skills. Alongside each Growing Need is a complementary Guiding Needs, the way *you* show up as a parent.

It helps to picture these as a duet. Your child's Growing Needs are one voice; your Guiding Needs are the harmony. When your steady presence offers Co-Regulation, their calm begins to grow. When you bring Body Respect, it reinforces their ability to trust their own body. When you practice Attunement, it supports not just one Need but all of them because nothing here works in isolation, every Guiding Need supports every Growing Need.

Growing Need	Guiding Need
Felt Safety: Knowing they are safe and cared for	**Attunement:** Noticing your child's unique signals and responding with sensitivity
Co-Regulation: Borrowing your calm when their big feelings take over	**Calm + Steady Presence:** Holding space when things feel messy
Body Trust: Learning to notice and believe their own hunger, fullness, and comfort signals	**Body Respect:** Showing your child, through your words and actions, that everyBODY deserves care

And you don't have to meet every Need every time. Sometimes you'll lose your calm. Sometimes you'll miss a cue. That's normal. Food Positivity isn't about perfection; it's about repair and returning to connection. Each small, steady moment adds up.

> ### "But What If I Lose My Calm?"
> That's normal. Every parent does. What matters most is connecting back, offering a hug, a smile, or a calm moment later. Repair teaches just as much if not more than getting it "right" in the first place.

Growing Skills ↔ Guiding Skills

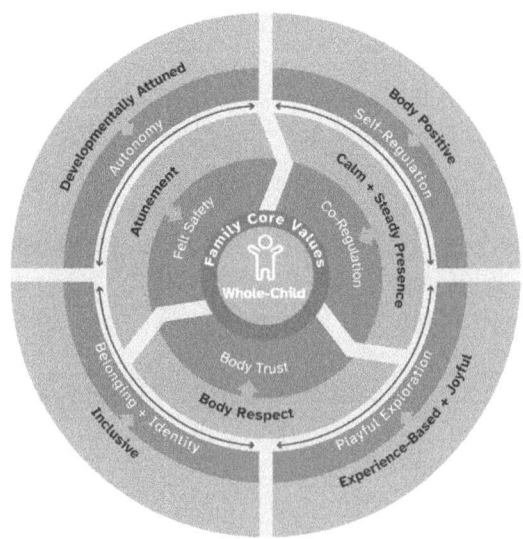

As kids grow, they're not just getting taller or learning new facts; they're building the life skills that they will carry with them into adulthood. Your role as the parent is to nurture these through your Guiding Skills.

Just like with Needs, each Guiding Skill has a complementary Growing Skill, but the magic is that they overlap and support one another. When you guide with Joy, it sparks Exploration *and* builds Belonging. When you stay Developmentally Attuned, it helps with Self-Regulation *and* Autonomy. Everything here works together, all Guiding Skills, supports all Growing Skills.

Growing Skill	Guiding Skill
Autonomy: Having a voice and making choices	**Developmentally Attuned:** Meeting your child where they are, not where you wish they were
Self-Regulation: Tuning into hunger, fullness, and feelings	**Body Positive:** Showing respect and kindness for all bodies, starting with your own
Playful Exploration: Learning through curiosity and discovery	**Experience-Based + Joyful:** Letting kids learn by doing, with play at the center
Belonging + Identity: Knowing they matter and are accepted	**Inclusive:** Making sure every child, every food, and every culture has a place at the table

You won't always be attuned or joyful in every moment. But small, steady practice adds up to help your child grow. They need presence, guidance, and room to try.

> **"What If My Child Resists or Doesn't Seem to Build These Skills?"**
>
> That's okay. Growth isn't a straight line. Some skills take longer, and some kids need more support. Keep offering opportunities, keep showing up, and keep meeting kids where they are—these tiny seeds you plant now take time to grow.

The Invisible Curriculum of the 3 Ms: Modeling, Messaging, and Moments

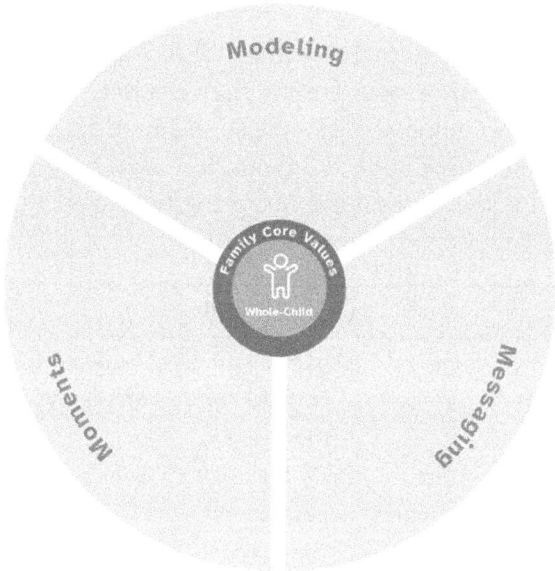

Surrounding all of these layers is the environment, the part that's always in the background.

Think of the environment as the background music of your child's life. Even if you're not actively teaching, the soundtrack is playing. It influences how safe they feel, how much they trust, and how curious they are to explore.

- **Modeling** is what your child sees. How you show kindness and care to your own body, how you try new foods, how you handle stress. Kids notice far more than we think.
- **Messaging** is what your child hears. How you talk about your own body, whether you call something "junk" or describe how it tastes, whether you talk about exercise as punishment or play.
- **Moments** are what your child experiences. The tone at the dinner table, the joy of baking together, the comfort of being allowed to say, "No, thank you."

It's about the little things you do, over and over. Sitting down together when you can. Choosing words that build trust. Letting your child know they're welcome at the table, exactly as they are.

"But What If I've Already Said the Wrong Thing or Modeled the Wrong Behavior?"

We're perfectly imperfect humans. Think about it as steady, imperfect practice. When you shift your words, when you explain, when you tell them you learned something new, when you say, "I wish I hadn't said that," you're teaching resilience and honesty—powerful lessons in themselves.

Food Positivity Life Skills

When you nurture your child's Needs and Skills, something lasting begins to grow—the Life Skills they'll carry with them long after childhood.

Growing Skills are part of the learning stage and Life Skills are the everyday habits, attitudes, and confidence that become second nature. And that's what makes Food Positivity more than just an approach to feeding. It's the lasting ability to relate to food and bodies with safety, trust, and joy.

In real life, Food Positivity looks like:

- Enjoying food without guilt, shame, or pressure
- Respecting that everyBODY and every food belongs
- Taking pride in your own cultural foods while honoring others'
- Questioning outside messages and checking them against your values

And it doesn't stop at the table. These everyday lessons carry into bigger life skills like self-awareness, emotional regulation, problem-solving, and resilience. Research shows these skills are protective, giving kids the confidence and compassion to handle a noisy world while staying connected to themselves and respectful of others.

"How Can I Model These Skills When I'm Still Working on Unlearning Old Diet Culture Messages Myself?"

The best way is to be honest. Let your child see that you're learning too. Saying things like "I'm practicing listening to my body" or "I'm learning how to be kinder to myself" shows them that growth is lifelong. You don't have to be perfect; practicing out loud is an incredible teaching tool that may be one of the most powerful lessons you can give them.

Research Spotlight: The Science of Flourishing

You've probably noticed that Food Positivity feels like more than just food. That's because it is.

Researchers in the field of positive psychology study what helps people *flourish*—not just survive, but truly thrive. One of the most well-known models is called PERMA, developed by psychologist Martin Seligman. PERMA describes five building blocks of well-being:

- **Positive Emotion:** Experiencing joy, curiosity, gratitude
- **Engagement:** Getting absorbed in an activity, like play or discovery
- **Relationships:** Feeling connected, safe, and valued
- **Meaning:** Having purpose and feeling part of something bigger
- **Accomplishment:** Building confidence through small wins

Sound familiar? That's because Food Positivity naturally gives kids *all five*.

- When mealtimes are pressure-free and playful, kids feel **joy**.
- When they knead dough, sniff herbs, or build snack "robots," they're deeply **engaged**.
- When family meals feel safe and inclusive, they strengthen **relationships**.

- When food connects to stories, science, or culture, kids discover **meaning**.
- And when they learn to trust their bodies or master a new skill, they feel a sense of **accomplishment**.

PERMA shows us that what you're practicing with Food Positivity isn't just good for meals—it's laying the foundation for lifelong well-being. You're not only raising kids who enjoy food and trust their bodies. You're raising kids who flourish.

The Food Positivity Protective Shield

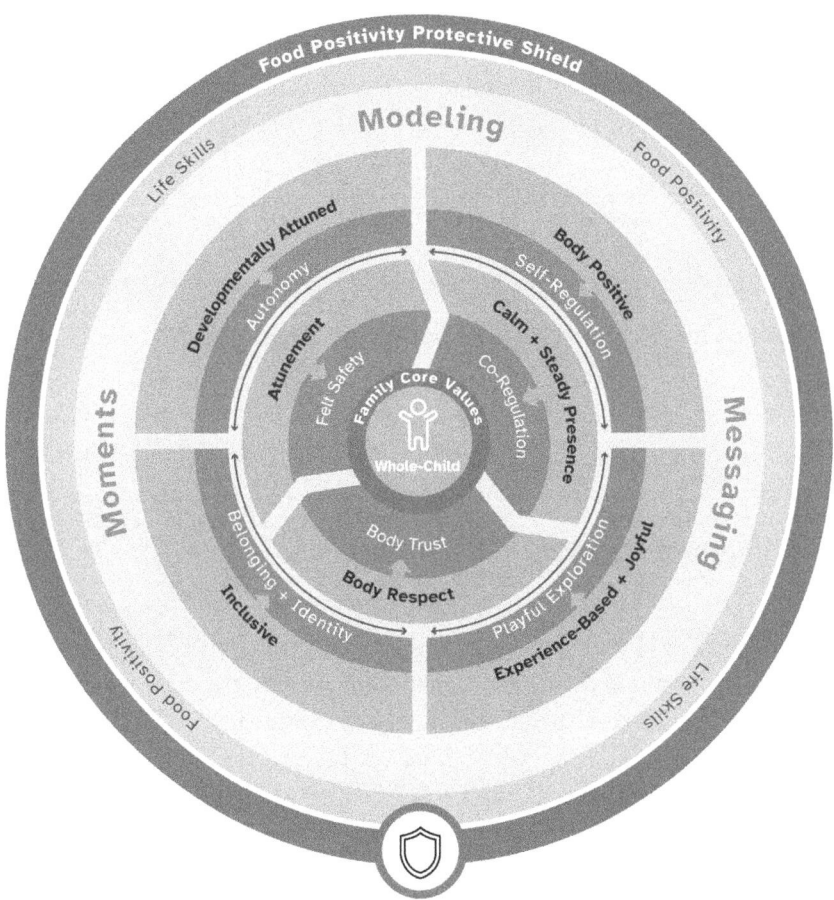

**Bonus Handout via the QR Code:** The Food Positivity Framework

When all of these layers work together with your steady guidance, a powerful Food Positivity Protective Shield begins to form.

The Protective Shield is your child's inner filter. It's the quiet, steady voice that helps them trust their body and question outside messages instead of accepting them as truth.

This shield doesn't block out diet culture completely. No shield can. Kids will still hear things from friends, teachers, media, and even doctors that don't align with your values. But instead of taking those messages in as truth, the shield helps them pause and sort: _Does this fit with what I know about myself? Does this match the values my family has taught me?_

That pause makes all the difference. Over time, the shield grows stronger, moment by moment, through the ordinary ways you show up: honoring hunger, letting "no thank you" be safe, speaking kindly about bodies, and creating joyful food experiences.

The goal isn't raising kids who never struggle. The world is too loud for that. The goal is raising kids who have a strong enough shield to come back to themselves, even when the noise outside gets overwhelming.

> **"But What If Diet Culture Still Gets Through?"**
> It will. That's part of growing up. The point isn't to make your child immune, but to give them the tools to filter what they hear and return to their own inner voice.

A Glimpse of Real Life

So what does all of this actually look like on a regular Tuesday?

At breakfast, you set out a couple of options and let your child choose. It's a small thing, but that choice gives them practice with autonomy and starts the day with a sense of confidence.

Before leaving the house you invite them to get hands-on as they help pack their own lunch, which is Experience-Based + Joyful.

Late afternoon, your child says, "I'm hungry," even though they had an afterschool snack two hours ago. Instead of brushing it off, you listen. You slice an apple, add some peanut butter, and talk about adding more food to their usual afternoon snack, checking in with how their body feels. That simple moment builds Body Trust.

At dinner, you serve food family-style and let your child scoop what they want, even if it's mostly bread tonight. With that choice, they practice Self-Regulation and Belonging, knowing their voice matters at the table.

None of these moments is perfect. They're ordinary and often messy, but they add up. Each is a thread in the bigger picture, weaving trust and confidence into your child's relationship with food.

The Tools You Need, Right Now

These shifts take time. It's normal to feel wobbly and lean on support while you practice. As long as you keep coming back to your values and your child's needs, you're making progress in supporting your child.

For now, it's also normal to need a little support. Feeding stirs up so many emotions—it's easy to feel caught off guard or unsure of what to say. That doesn't mean you're doing it wrong; it just means you're human, still working out how to show up for your child.

That's where the scripts in the next part come in. Think of them as training wheels, not the exact right thing to say. They're rooted in the ideas you've been learning so far, so the words you lean on stay aligned with the kind of connection and leadership you want to bring to the table. They'll give you a place to start when emotions at the table are running high or when your child asks a question you weren't prepared for.

And just like training wheels, you won't need them forever. With practice, you'll begin to find words that feel natural and true to *you*, grounded in *your* Family Core Values and *your* child's needs. In time, your instincts will take the lead, and you'll step fully into your role as a confident Food Leader raising kids with Food Positivity.

Bringing It Home

This is the heart of Food Positivity: raising a child who feels safe, seen, and supported. A child who knows they can trust their body, who feels at home at the table, and who carries a sense of confidence with them out into the world.

And here's the reminder we hope you carry with you: all of this is about growth and learning. There is no such thing as perfection or doing it "right." There will be days you lose your calm, serve cereal for dinner, or wish you'd said something differently.

Every time you offer a choice, honor your child's cue, or create a joyful moment, you're building something bigger than the meal in front of you. You're shaping how your child will feel about food and their body for years to come. You're planting seeds of trust, one ordinary moment at a time.

The full framework may feel like a lot, but it's not here for you to follow like a checklist. It's here to open your mind and your heart to navigate a better way forward for your child and raise them with the experiences you never had.

You don't have to do this alone, and you don't have to figure it out from scratch. You have the map, and next, you'll have the words.

One Simple Step

Pick one everyday food interaction and ask yourself, "What seed am I planting here?" Whether it's letting your child serve themselves or eat an unlimited amount of a food that scares you to practice Self-Regulation or modeling Body Respect yourself, you're supporting their Food Positivity for life, one small step at a time.

Your Food Positivity Practice

Mapping Your Four Foundations

PART

IV

Scripts and Strategies for Compassionate Conversations

15

How to Talk to Kids About Food (Without Shame or Fear)

My daughter asks for snacks constantly, and I never know how to respond. If I say no, I worry she'll think I'm restricting her. But if I always say yes, I'm afraid she'll fill up on snacks instead of meals. I usually try stalling with "maybe later" or "let's just wait for dinner," but even that feels like I'm dismissing her needs. And I never know if she's actually hungry, or maybe just bored. I just want her to enjoy food without either of us overthinking it!

—Kimberly

EVERYTHING LEADING UP to this point has been designed to help you understand where the confusion around talking to kids about food comes from, how children absorb the messages we send, and what it truly means to take responsibility for feeding them well—both nutritionally and emotionally.

Now, it's time to get practical. Let's walk through the most common food-related scenarios we hear about from parents and offer compassionate scripts and strategies to help you navigate them. As you read, notice how each strategy and script supports your child's Growing Needs and Growing Skills and how they ask *you* to use your Guiding Needs, Guiding Skills, and the 3 Ms.

You're the G.U.I.D.E.

All along, you've been learning that you are your child's trusted Food Leader. And this role goes far beyond what you serve. You're *guiding* your child through the process of everything they need to build Food Positivity.

A huge part of Food Positivity is saying "yes" to our children's desires about food when it makes sense. Yes to exploration, to joyful experiences, and to the foods they most enjoy. But for logistical and nutritional reasons, you simply won't be able to say "yes" all of the time. And as we saw in Chapter 12, feeling frustrated when things don't go exactly how they want and learning to cope with that frustration is an important element of your child developing Self-Regulation and growing into a well-adjusted adult.

Let's look at how you can use your Guiding Needs to support your child through frustrating food situations when your answer needs to be "no." Our **G.U.I.D.E.** tool will help you put these skills into practice in a way that supports your individual child.

> **Scenario:** Your child wants an energy bar, but they're pricey, and it aligns with your Family Core Value of financial stewardship to reserve them as a convenient option for sports practice.

G—Give acknowledgment: Start by recognizing and affirming your child's experience. Here, you are practicing Attunement. By noticing and reflecting what your child is experiencing back to them, you show them that you heard and understood their request.

"You'd like an energy bar right now."

U—Uplift their request: Honoring your child's desire, even when you can't grant it, is how you practice Body Respect. This affirms that their desires and body signals are real and meaningful. You don't dismiss their desire (e.g., "You don't need that right now"). You acknowledge the fact that it makes sense in *their* internal world, and there is nothing inherently wrong with that, which takes shame out of the equation. Sharing your own aligned perspective brings in empathy, another protection against shame.

"That would be really yummy. I wish we could enjoy them all the time too. . ."

I—Introduce the limit: Here is where you bring in your Calm and Steady Presence. Calmly state your limit. You're not snapping or replying with exasperation, (e.g., "Quit asking me!"), but you're not being permissive either. As the Food Leader, you're holding steady to the limit you've determined is in your child's best interest, rooted in your Family Core Values.

". . .but we're not having one right now because we really do need to save them for soccer practice."

Note that the degree to which you explain your reasoning will depend on your child's age. To a very young child, you might simply end with "We're not having one right now" because making rational decisions about the future is beyond their understanding. To an older child, you might add "Because they cost more than our other snacks" because they're beginning to have an understanding of money.

D—Describe and support their struggle: Naming emotions like frustration, disappointment, or sadness communicates, "I understand what's happening inside you." You suggest an emotion they might be feeling through your Attunement and help them work through it via your Calm and Steady Presence. This process helps children recognize and label their emotions. Offering support for your child to work through this struggle helps them build a set of tools to eventually work through these difficult feelings on their own (Co-regulation → Self-Regulation).

"It looks like you're feeling frustrated. Is that right? Do you want to (tell me more about it/take some deep breaths/do some jumping jacks)?"

E—End with options: Once you've made your limit clear, you offer a realistic, positive alternative aligned with your child's needs. If it is meal or snack time or your Attunement tells you that your child is genuinely hungry, this can be another item you'll serve. If it's not time to eat, you can identify exactly when you *will* serve the item and/or suggest another activity to focus on. This again demonstrates Body Respect while maintaining your role as the Food Leader.

"Let's have some of these cookies with our snack instead" and/or "We'll definitely have an energy bar at soccer practice."

Let's take a look at two more examples:

> **Scenario:** Your child is not yet old enough to make the connection between what they're eating and an immediate physical consequence, such as citrus causing diaper rash. You choose to limit the food because of your Family Core Values of safety and well-being.

"More oranges would be delicious, but we're all done with oranges right now. It's okay to be sad! Would you like some apples, or do you just want to keep eating your mac and cheese?"

Note that this type of decision works best if the consequence is something that's definitely happened in the past, not what you're worried might happen. And the older a child grows and has the opportunity to practice Self-Regulation, the more you can trust them to make these sorts of decisions for themselves.

> **Scenario:** Your child doesn't want to share the food available from a communal dish or wants so much that there wouldn't be enough for others:

"I know you love mashed potatoes, but that bowl is for the whole family. Let's have one scoop each, and you can have this meatloaf, broccoli, and your cookie too. I can see you're disappointed. I'll make sure to make even more potatoes next time!"

But How Do You Tell the Difference?

Another concern we so often hear is that parents are unsure when they should say "yes" versus when they should say "no," especially when it comes to nutrition-related decisions. And while it sure would be convenient if we could give you a list of firm "yes" and "no" situations, there's simply no such thing.

Think of it this way: You probably don't feel guilty or unsure about holding firm to your child's scheduled bedtime on a school night, even if they beg to stay up for another hour. You know that getting enough rest supports your Family Core Value of well-being and declining that request is in their best interest. But you might just as easily let your child stay up late on a fun Friday night, because it supports your values of connection and joy.

Your decision is always rooted in your values, even when it results in different actions depending on the situation.

Remember, guilt is the feeling of making decisions that are *not* aligned with our values. And feeling unsure about *what* to decide is probably a sign that you're not yet confident in the values guiding your decisions. Or you may have more learning to do about what your child truly needs to be well. That's okay! These are just signs that you need to do a little more reflection to nail down this process.

What You Can Always Say

Before we dive into how to address specific scenarios, we want you to have a few phrases you can always say in response to your child's questions about food.

Special Note: If your child struggles with ARFID, PFD, failure to thrive or any other specific condition that results in low food intake or limited variety, we encourage you *not* to emphasize "Our bodies need all different kinds of food." In those cases, the first priority is the child getting *enough* total food, regardless of the variety (on the advice of your medical team, of course). Instead you can say, "I'm here to help you get the food you need."

You're the Food Leader, and it's helpful to share with your child what this means in terms they can understand, just like you do with your other responsibilities, like keeping them safe and going to work. You can always say:

"Our bodies need all different kinds of food."

Keep in mind that this statement should never be used to pressure the child to eat certain foods (e.g., "You need to eat some vegetables because our bodies need all different kinds of food"). It's simply to explain your reasoning for what you have and haven't chosen to serve at any given meal or snack. This statement supports your Family Core Value of well-being without introducing age-inappropriate nutrition concepts. It's the same as saying "Our bodies need to rest" when it's time for bed without getting into the specifics of sleep science.

Another phrase that will help you is:

"It's my job to serve your meals, and it's your job to choose which of those foods you want to eat."

This explains the Division of Responsibility in a child-friendly way and emphasizes your role as the trustworthy Food Leader. By making these roles clear—especially to a young child—you support their Growing Needs. You reassure them that you will always provide the food they need (Felt Safety), you will stay steady and predictable while they learn about food and feelings (Co-Regulation), and they can always listen to their own hunger, fullness, and preferences (Body Trust).

So keep those statements in the back of your mind as you read through the following scenarios.

Scripts and Scenarios

As always, there's no one-size-fits-all response! The best approach will depend on your Attunement to your child and your understanding of what might be driving their behavior. Think of these scripts as starting points, not word-for-word recommendations. We encourage you to adapt them to your voice, your values, and, most importantly, your child's unique needs.

Let's start with a few strategies you can use in many different scenarios. Relying on these particular strategies will actually nip many other food struggles in the bud by meeting your child's needs, building trust, and quite literally filling their bodies with the calories they need to avoid a dysregulated meltdown.

Strategy: Regular Meals and Snacks

This one is not news to you by now, but it's so important we'll say it one last time. When your child trusts that you will regularly provide the food they need—and enjoy—it promotes Felt Safety and builds trust that their Food Leader will always provide for them. This is also your best tool to stay ahead of "hangry" meltdowns, which often lead to other issues. Regular meals also expose kids to variety and help them arrive at the table with an appetite for the balanced meal you've planned and practice Self-Regulation. Of course, it's especially helpful to serve at least one preferred/safe food at each eating occasion, if not more.

Strategy: Match Meals to Hunger Patterns

Yes, you're responsible for "when" food is served, but it's not fair to your child that they should have to wait until an arbitrary, predetermined time for the meal. Use your Attunement to figure out when your child is most hungry over the course of a typical day and plan meals and snacks for these times.

Of course, the logistics of this get tricky at times! If the meal you're planning takes an hour to cook but your kid is starving as soon as they get home from school, what's a parent to do? You can prepare food in advance if time allows, but this is also a great time to lean on nutrient-dense convenience foods, many of which are heat-and-eat.

Strategy: Check Regulation First

Through your Attunement, consider whether your child is tired, upset, overstimulated, or too hungry to focus. Meeting those needs *first* will make mealtimes smoother. Note that you don't always have to talk about this. You can simply decide to grab a snack or postpone the meal for a few minutes to handle the situation. Or you can say:

> "I wonder if you're feeling [emotion] right now. I have an idea. Let's [activity that supports your child's need]."

Strategy: Connection Outside of Mealtimes

Sometimes, a situation entirely unrelated to food has your child feeling anxious or unsure, which shows up at the table in their eating patterns. And sometimes, they just need a little more connection with *you*, their trusted grown-up. Spend time with your child playing, reading, or using your Calm and Steady Presence to talk through whatever is going on with them, and you may just find that battles at the table naturally subside.

Strategy: Use Positive Language

One of our favorites, we love positivity! Using positive language about *all* food is your best tool to avoid creating unintended food hierarchies, which often break our child's trust and lead to shame. Because if we're excited about "broccoli trees" but reserved or simply neutral about cookies and ice cream, our kids will catch on to our agenda that we're more invested in them eating the one we're hyping up. Try:

> "I bought some of those gummy candies you were asking about! I'm excited to try the different flavors. We'll have them with dinner tonight."
>
> "Check out how these peppers come in all different colors! Isn't it cool how they grow like this?"

But be careful not to use these statements in a coded, "Don't you wanna try it?" kind of way, as that can come off as pressure. And for particularly hesitant kids, it helps to match your enthusiasm to their comfort level. That sounds like this:

"There will be lots of different foods at the barbeque today. Burgers, veggies, cupcakes. I'll help you make a plate of food that looks good to you."

And here's an important tip: Teach your kids to use kind words about food. This includes "Don't yuck my yum" (aka not saying negative things about a food someone else enjoys). But it's also about treating food with respect. Someone took care to grow it, someone else took care to prepare it, and it nourishes the many people who enjoy it. Here's how you can help your kids learn this skill:

"I heard you say Grandma's lasagna is disgusting. It's perfectly okay to say you don't like it or it's not for you, but please remember to use kind words about food."

Talking to Your Child About Food Requests

We *know* you struggle with this. And because our kids' curiosity about food is so important to Playful Exploration, we want them to know it's always okay for them to ask about it. But as the Food Leader, it is also your job to ensure that the food available to your kids meets their needs until they fully develop the Self-Regulation to do so themselves. Sometimes that's pausing for an impromptu snack, and other times it's declining their requests.

> **Scenario:** Your child asks for food between planned meals and snacks.

Always use "Check Regulation First" when your child requests food between planned meals. If they're genuinely hungry, pause for a quick snack. This is also a time to reflect on "Match Meal Patterns to Hunger" and use your Attunement to figure out whether there's any reason your kid is not eating quite enough at the meals you're serving. And even if your child *is* hungry, you don't have to grant the request for exactly what they're asking for (although that's also an option).

Strategy: "Let's Have It Soon"

If it's not the right time to eat what they're asking about, reassuring your child that you'll serve their requested food at a future meal balances structure with Attunement. It also helps you maintain your responsibilities as the Food Leader and meet the request at a time that makes sense in terms of both logistics and nutrition. Kids learn their preferences matter to you, even when you can't say yes right away. You can communicate this with G.U.I.D.E.:

> "Those cupcakes look good, huh? They are for dessert, and we're having pretzels and hummus for snack today. It's not quite snack time yet, but I can see you're hungry so let's have it early. Hey, when we have dessert later, do you want a chocolate or vanilla cupcake?"

And when they say, *"But I want one right now!"* stick with G.U.I.D.E.:

> "I hear you. They look delicious! Remember, it's my job to serve you all different kinds of foods, so right now we're having pretzels. Would you like to read this book with me while we sit at the table?"

Scenario: Your child didn't eat much of the meal and asks for snacks soon after.

We get it. It's reasonable to think, "If you weren't hungry for dinner, how could you possibly be hungry for snacks?" But this is a missed opportunity to demonstrate Attunement to your child's needs. Reflect on what they're likely communicating to you with this request. Often when kids are asking for snacks outside of scheduled meals, it's because persistent requests are the only time they actually get those foods or because they *are* genuinely hungry but the foods or food environment at the table didn't feel safe enough to them.

Strategy: Preferred Foods Often

This is a little different from simply including a "safe" food with the meal. This is constructing meals *mainly* from the foods your child most enjoys, with perhaps an item or two they don't like yet. It communicates your Attunement to their preferences and helps them see the table as a place that meets their need for Felt Safety, where they won't be pressured or overwhelmed by unfamiliar foods. You don't have to do this indefinitely, but it can be a helpful "starter" strategy when you're first shifting toward the Food Positivity approach. As your child's comfort level at the table increases, you can change up the ratio of preferred foods to new or less-preferred options, again using your Attunement to determine when they are up for the challenge. Try inviting your child to the table like this:

> "Hey, I've been thinking. I really want you to enjoy your meals with me. I'm thinking of switching up what I cook, any requests? I also noticed that you've been asking for potato chips often, so I thought we could include those as a side dish sometimes."

Another reason kids commonly ask for snacks after dinner is that the timing of the meal didn't line up with their hunger patterns. And while "Match Meals to Hunger Patterns" is helpful, it's not always possible, especially at dinner. So try:

Strategy: Planned Bedtime Snack

This is a filling snack you plan into your bedtime routine. Scheduling this snack rather than caving to snack requests or insisting that dinner is their last opportunity for food both helps you match your child's hunger patterns to their opportunities to eat and gives you a place to direct "Let's Have it Soon." Also keep in mind that this snack can certainly include what they're asking for, but as the Food Leader you can also offer other items to add balance. This food doesn't have to be complicated—think cereal, yogurt, cheese, fruit, etc. Explain when the bedtime snack will be with G.U.I.D.E.:

> "You're asking for popcorn, I hear you. We just finished dinner so right now I need to clean up and it's time for you to read. We'll have a snack again right before bed. I'm planning popcorn, milk and apple slices."

Scenario: Your child frequently asks for sweets.

This is one of the most common questions we get! You don't want your child to feel like sweets are off-limits, but you also know they can't thrive on sugar alone.

Strategy: One Portion of Dessert with Dinner

Serving dessert right along with dinner can make sweets feel like a normal part of eating, not something extra or off-limits. This strategy is often shared as part of Ellyn Satter's Division of Responsibility. Children can eat the dessert whenever they like, which keeps them from rushing through the meal just to get to dessert. But it's limited to one portion so that the child still has a chance to consume nutrients from the other foods available at the meal.

You can explain why a second portion isn't available with G.U.I.D.E.:

"Those cookies sure are yummy! At dinner we just have one cookie because our bodies need all different kinds of food. It's okay to be disappointed. We still have rice, chicken, and carrots. We'll have dessert again tomorrow."

And when your child inevitably replies with, *"I want another cookie now!"* just hold your boundary:

"I know you do. It's okay to be frustrated. We'll have more cookies tomorrow."

Remember, the more consistent you are with meeting your child's Growing Needs, the more they'll learn to trust your "no." But this is also a two-pronged strategy. If dessert is *sometimes* limited to one portion, it's *also* important to offer:

Strategy: Unlimited Favorites at Planned Times

Create opportunities for your child to enjoy as much of the sweets they love as their body wants. This can be a planned snack or after-dinner dessert and these occasions often naturally arise at holidays or special events. The goal is to help your child practice their Growing Skill of Self-Regulation, noticing how different amounts of food feel so they can start figuring out what's right for them next time.

You don't have to say much about this strategy other than:

"Let's have as many cookies as we want with this snack!" or "Of course you can have another cupcake!" at a celebration (assuming there's enough for everyone).

And yes, sometimes they will eat so much of the sweets that they don't feel well. This is experience-based learning and it's part of the process! We'll talk about supporting your child through these body sensations in the next chapter.

> **Scenario:** Your child wants something completely different from what you've served.

This is a normal part of your child testing out their Growing Skill of Autonomy. But if you're confident that you did your job of putting together a meal including foods they enjoy, you don't have to be a short-order cook. But often, food refusals—especially of foods your child typically enjoys—stem from something emotional rather than actually wanting something different. If your Attunement tells you this might be the case, try:

Strategy: "Would You Like to Add"

If your child's refusal might be stemming from a heightened need for Autonomy (no matter how well you did your job of planning a meal you thought they'd enjoy) use your "what" responsibility of DOR to grant one more addition to the meal. Note that this shouldn't involve you cooking anything new. Using G.U.I.D.E., try:

"I can see you're not excited about this pasta. That's okay! I'm not cooking anything else right now, but if you'd like to pick either strawberries or yogurt from the fridge, go ahead. I'm here to help you find what works."

Often, this small nod to their need for Autonomy will even help kids relax enough to start eating the other elements of the meal, too. But another option is not adding any more food to the meal via the "Let's Have It Soon" strategy. Of course we want our kids to be confident in speaking up about the foods they enjoy, but it's not always practical to do so. Your Attunement will help you make that choice.

Supporting Your Child When You Have Concerns About Their Nutrition

This is the top concern among the parents we work with! A lot of this concern stems from the confusing messages about "healthy" diets we all absorb from diet culture. Consult Chapter 6 to help cut through the noise and learn more about what your child *really* needs. Also consider a chat with your pediatrician or even an evaluation with a registered dietitian trained in responsive feeding to put your mind at ease and help you understand areas of your child's diet that may need more attention.

Also note that we're *not* providing scripts or strategies to help you *convince* your child to eat what they need. As we've seen, it's just not developmentally appropriate for young kids and it doesn't demonstrate Body Respect. It's *your* job as the Food Leader to find ways to meet your child's needs, not *their* job to understand nutrition.

> **Scenario:** Your child wants the same food every day and resists variety

As we covered in Chapter 13, it's okay for kids to have their preferences! At the same time, it's also your responsibility as the Food Leader to do what you can to help them feel comfortable with a variety of foods. You can try:

Strategy: Gentle Exposure

Seeing food again and again in a no-pressure way promotes your child's sense of Felt Safety with the food. Research shows that this slow and steady approach is how most kids warm up to new foods. Remember that exposure doesn't mean *eating* the food or even having it on their plate. It can be just being near the food and watching others eat it.

Strategy: Modeling Variety Yourself

Recall from the 3 Ms that kids are always learning from our actions. Modeling consumption of the same variety of foods you hope your child will grow to enjoy teaches them that these foods are safe and might even be delicious! This happens even if you never say a word about what you're eating, but you can also narrate your experience, such as:

> "Hmm, I've never tried roasted cauliflower before, but I know I like raw cauliflower. Let me see how this is different."

Also try: "Preferred Foods Often" and the food exploration strategies in Chapter 17.

Scenario: Your child doesn't seem to be eating a balanced diet.

Strategy: Growing Needs Come Before Nutrition

As we learned in Chapter 5, meeting your child's Growing Needs has to come *before* quality nutrition or even their ability to practice Self-Regulation. This means that there *will* be times where their diet isn't perfectly aligned with nutrition recommendations while you focus on supporting their Growing Needs.

"Preferred Foods Often" and "Unlimited Favorites at Planned Times" align well with this strategy. The goal, of course, is that once you're supporting their Growing Needs well, they have enough opportunities to practice their Growing Skills and begin to regulate their dietary patterns on their own.

Strategy: Nutrition Through Preferred Foods

If your child is truly lacking in a nutrient, the best way for them to get it is via food they enjoy. Sure, milk is a great source of calcium, but if your child doesn't like it, then pressuring them to drink it or guilting them for not compromises Felt Safety—no matter how positively you frame their need for it. Get creative on how else you can add the nutrient by serving more of foods they like and introducing new options aligned with their tastes. You don't actually have to say anything about this, but if you want to you can say:

> "Hey, I noticed you don't like milk much. That's no big deal. Since our bodies need all different kinds of foods, I was thinking I could serve yogurt more often. Which flavor should I get?"

Strategy: Use Supplements Thoughtfully

Supplements are a great option to fill in true nutrition gaps while you work toward helping your child feel comfortable and relaxed enough to get what they need through food. Some foods are fortified, like orange juice with calcium, and options like gummy vitamins and fiber powders can help too. Just make sure to consult a health professional to confirm whether your child has a true need for the nutrient and the product you select is safe. You can say:

> "I was talking to your pediatrician, and she told me that you need a little extra of this nutrient called calcium. These calcium chews are kinda like medicine for that, but they're chocolate flavored! I'll give you one every morning with breakfast."

> **Scenario:** Your child wants more of an item that would negatively impact their nutrition

Another part of your job as the Food Leader is to gently limit items that would indeed have a big impact on your child's overall diet quality. This is why the information in Chapter 6 is so critical. You can't accurately make these decisions if you don't know what your child genuinely needs! But diet culture can make that *really* hard to actually determine. When you're confident that more of a certain food is simply too much and your child doesn't yet have the Self-Regulation skills to figure this out for themselves, you can use:

Strategy: Gentle Limits on One Food with Other Options Available

As the Food Leader, you know the specifics of the nutrition your child needs, but only *they* know how much feels right for their body. Some days they'll eat much less than you expect, and other days they'll surprise you with how much they want. Both are normal! In cases where the particular item they are eating will truly result in an overall nutritional imbalance, use your Calm and Steady Presence and G.U.I.D.E. to say:

> "I know you'd love some more milk, but we've had three cups today already, so that's not what I'm serving right now. We still have plenty of strawberries and cookies for you to enjoy."

You can absolutely use this strategy with sweets and snacks, too. When the food is something your child is particularly fixated on, we also recommend pairing the limit with "Unlimited Favorites at Planned Times," which sounds like this:

> "I know you love chocolate! We're just having three pieces with lunch today, but you still have your sandwich and crackers. How about we pick one day this week to eat as much as we want after school?"

These strategies combined help *you* help your child get the nutrition they need while also creating opportunities to practice Self-Regulation. Remember that in these moments, the key is always that your child trusts you to make these decisions on their behalf, because of how well you have met their Growing Needs. It's a "with great power comes great responsibility" type of situation! They will likely still be frustrated, and that's okay too.

EXPERT INSIGHT: Navigating Conversations About Disordered Eating

Zoë Bisbing, LCSW, psychotherapist, eating disorder specialist, and creator of Body-Positive Home

If you're truly concerned, that your child's eating habits may be signs of an eating disorder, it's important to navigate the conversation with care.

(continued)

(*continued*)

Scenario: You suspect your child may be engaging in disordered eating or showing signs of an eating disorder.

It's frightening to suspect your child may be restricting food to change their body. Parents often swing toward two extremes: the *alarmist*, who panics and says, "Just eat," or the *avoider*, who notices something is off but hopes it will pass. Both come from love, but neither makes kids feel safe. Instead, try approaching with these 5Cs:

Calm—Set the tone. Choose a quiet, nonmeal moment—driving in the car, walking the dog, or during a moment of downtime.

Curious—Explore without judgment. Say, "Hey, I've noticed you've been skipping dessert/eating less/reading labels a lot/asking a lot about what's in the food I'm preparing. Have you noticed this too?" It's normal to get a shrug or minimal response. This stuff is extremely hard to talk about, but you show you are not afraid and are able to support them when you lead this way.

Concerned—Name the concern clearly. "Sometimes these behaviors can be signs that someone's having a hard time." It is typical that the child or teen will not share your concern, but that does not mean your concern isn't valid.

Connect—Reinforce love and presence. "I care about you, and I'm here to help."

Confident—Signal support and next steps. "If this feels hard to talk about or to change, that's okay—we'll get help together."

And then, Consultation. It isn't wise to wait too long before seeking professional input. The first step is often a parent consultation with a mental health eating disorder specialist. That initial meeting can be parent-only, giving you space to share observations and map out next steps. Early support is essential for long-term well-being and safety, and you don't need to navigate this alone.

Bringing It Home

The more you practice Food Positivity, the more natural these conversations will feel. You're learning a new language, a way of talking about food that you never learned growing up yourself. The Food Positivity way. It takes time, but eventually you'll find yourself fluent, speaking with ease in ways that support your child's needs and strengthen their trust in the care you provide.

When you do second-guess yourself (and you will!), treat yourself with compassion and return to your Family Core Values for some clarity. They'll remind you why you chose this path and guide your next steps. Keep practicing, keep reflecting, and know that you are giving your child the gift of Food Positivity that lasts far beyond the table.

One Simple Step: Listen, Then Lead

Next time you're not sure what to say about food, call the G.U.I.D.E. tool to mind so you can address your child's needs in a supportive and empathetic way.

Your Food Positivity Practice

G.U.I.D.E. in Action

16

How to Talk About Bodies (So Kids Learn to Trust Theirs)

My daughter has started making little comments about her body, like asking if her stomach looks "too big" or if she should skip dessert. She's only nine. I tell her she's perfect as she is, but she doesn't seem convinced. Last week she stood in front of the mirror and tugged at her shirt. I tried to change the subject and make her laugh, but I could feel her pulling away. I don't want to make it worse by saying the wrong thing, but I'm terrified that she's going to have the same body image issues that I do.

—Natalia

WHEN YOU'VE STRUGGLED with Body Trust yourself, talking about bodies with kids can feel like walking through a minefield. When we didn't grow up hearing positive, affirming language about all bodies, we just don't feel like we have the language to "get it right" in the moment. But just like talking about food, these conversations will get easier with practice. The more you reflect on your values and show up with intention, the more natural this language will feel.

As you begin having these conversations, you may notice a common thread—one we've been building toward all along. Some of your body talk will be inward, helping your child notice what's happening in their own body: how hungry or full they feel, how certain foods affect them, or how their body changes as it grows and develops. Other times, the focus is outward, reflecting on how their body exists in relation to others and the diversity of bodies in the world around them.

But both kinds of conversations come back to your Guiding Need of Body Respect and Guiding Skill of Body Positive Learning. We want our kids to know that everyBODY deserves to be celebrated, understood, and treated with care. So whether your child is learning to trust what's happening inside their own body, unquestionably believing that their own body is good and worthy exactly as it is, or to see and speak about others with compassion, you're teaching them that all bodies are valuable just as they are.

Strategies You Can Use in Many Scenarios

Just like with food, these universal strategies help you show up with consistency and confidence, even when you feel caught off guard. They remind you to meet your child with openness, to model the kind of language you want them to internalize, and to keep the focus on their own body's signals and unique needs. When you use these strategies often, you reinforce the values of respect, compassion, and body trust that will guide your child for years to come.

Strategy: Use Positive Language About Bodies (Including Your Own)

Children learn how to value bodies through the 3 Ms. By choosing respectful, compassionate language—whether about their body, your own, or someone else's—you Model that all bodies are worthy of dignity. This doesn't mean ignoring your child's genuine challenges or frustrations with their body (or your own), but it does mean refusing to equate worth with appearance. This can sound like:

"My tummy is soft, and that's part of what makes me warm and huggable." "I really love how your eyes light up when you laugh!"

And if you're really struggling to say anything positive about your own body, that's okay. That is part of the trauma of growing up in a world that didn't accept you exactly as you are. You can lean on neutral language until you get there.

Strategy: Lead with Curiosity

When you prioritize Body Trust, Autonomy, and Body Positive learning, you help your child see that there's no wrong way to *have* a body and no wrong way to feel *in* a body. Curiosity is the tool that keeps conversations open. Instead of criticizing or fixing (e.g., "I told you if you ate that you'd get a stomachache" or "Next time, just eat slower"), you invite your child to share more about what they're noticing or feeling. This communicates that their experiences are valid and encourages them to use their own cues and emotions as guides in making sense of bodies. This applies both to physical sensations related to eating and body image concerns. It can sound like:

> "Hmm, what do you think your body (or emotions) is trying to tell you right now?"
>
> "Do you remember if you've ever felt like this before? What helped then?"

Another helpful strategy to support your child's need for Co-Regulation is to gently introduce your own experiences.

Strategy: Name and Normalize Sensations

Kids are constantly learning how to interpret and respond to the signals their bodies send, like hunger, fullness, excitement, or nervousness. But in a world that often overrides those cues (e.g., "Clean your plate" and "You can't be hungry, you just ate!"), learning to trust their body can feel confusing. By suggesting names for what they might be feeling—like hunger, fullness, tiredness, excitement, sadness—you help your child connect those sensations to language they can use to understand and work through their feelings in a healthy way as they develop Self-Regulation. And by normalizing those sensations, you teach your child that body signals aren't shameful—they're simply information to notice and learn from, which strengthens Body Trust.

> "I think what you're describing could be hunger. It doesn't always show up through a grumbling tummy, sometimes it feels like not having much energy or having trouble focusing. Could that be what you're feeling?"

Strategy: Share Your Own Experience

This strategy is *very* nuanced, because just because you do or don't feel a certain way, it doesn't mean your child will have the same experience. So what we're *not* looking for here is anything like "When I don't eat vegetables, I don't feel well" with the goal of *getting* the child to eat vegetables. The real goal is to support "Name and Normalize Sensations" with connection and empathy and suggest possible coping strategies that may become tools they rely on themselves in the future. This can sound like:

> "Sometimes when I eat too fast, I notice my stomach feels tight like that. Could that be what you're feeling right now? What I do is drink water and lie down until I feel better; should we try that?"
>
> "I've had times when I didn't like how my tummy looked too. It made me feel like I didn't fit in. When that happens to me, I try to think about all the great things my body can do, no matter how it looks. Is that how you feel, or is it something different for you?"

Body Sensations About Eating

Helping your child identify how different foods feel in their bodies—or the lack of food at all—is an important part of their need for Co-Regulation. Note that not every meal needs to be chock-full of body conversations. It's definitely okay to just *eat* most of the time! But you may find natural times to help them connect what they're eating.

> **Scenario:** Your child feels unwell, likely because of what they did or didn't eat

When your child shares something they feel or if your Attunement tells you something might be off, both "Lead with Curiosity," and "Name and Normalize Sensations" are your best tools for helping your child understand what's happening in their body and build awareness of their own Self-Regulation needs. It also helps to name the support you're offering through your Calm and Steady Presence.

Strategy: "I'm Here to Help You Feel Good in Your Body"

When your child feels uncomfortable or unsure about what their body is telling them, they need to know you're there to help. You likely know from experience that shaming doesn't help build positive habits (e.g., "It's because you're always eating so much sugar" or "I told you that you needed to eat more of your lunch"). Instead, your supportive words reassure your child that body sensations aren't something to feel bad about; they're information you can explore together. In the moment, that might mean helping your child rest, offering water, or simply sitting with them until they feel better—strategies you'll determine through "Lead with Curiosity." And it also means using what you've both learned to guide *your* future decisions as the Food Leader. You can say:

"I'm here to help you feel good in your body. Let's figure out what it might need right now."

By responding with care now *and* preparing with intention later, you show your child that their comfort and well-being are always part of the plan—exactly what they'll adopt for their own self-care habits as adults.

Scenario: Your child has overeaten and feels uncomfortable.

This is really no different from the previous scenario, but because of how diet culture teaches us that overeating is a shameful lack of self-control, we want to provide you with some extra support.

Start with the "Regular Meals and Snacks" strategy, since eating too little earlier in the day can lead to overeating later—it's the body's way of making sure it gets enough food (hello, binge eating). Still, your meal timing won't always be perfect, and other times food just tastes so good, your child won't want to stop eating. These moments are a normal part of learning Self-Regulation. To build on "Name and Normalize Sensations" and "I'm Here to Help You Feel Good in Your Body," you can try the following strategy.

Strategy: Normalize Overeating

Even people who are very skilled in Self-Regulation do it from time to time. For your child, overeating is a normal part of learning Self-Regulation and avoiding overeating (for the most part) down the line. When you frame overeating as a chance to learn about Body Trust and self-care, your child learns that feeling too full isn't something to feel ashamed of; it's just more information. You can help them reflect on what their body is telling with your Calm and Steady Presence by saying:

> "Sometimes our eyes want more than our tummy can hold. That's okay! Everyone feels that way sometimes. You'll get better at figuring out the right amount of food as you get older, and I'm always here to help you."

Also return to "Lead with Curiosity" and "Share Your Own Experience" to support your child in developing self-care skills to cope with feeling uncomfortable and more or less avoiding overeating in the future.

Scenario: Your child tends not to be hungry for a certain meal.

This is a common one, especially at breakfast given the fact that school and childcare schedules don't always allow for ideal use of "Match Meals to Hunger Patterns." But instead of pressuring your child to eat, you can try the following strategy.

Strategy: Bring It Back to *Their* Body

Every child's body has its own rhythms, signals, and needs. When you gently guide your child to notice what their body is telling them—hunger, fullness, comfort, discomfort, or growth—you support Body Trust and Self-Regulation through curiosity and awareness. This teaches them that their body is worth listening to and caring for, just as it is. So instead of saying what you assume will happen (e.g., "You're going to be starving until lunch if you don't eat!"), you can say:

> "Do you remember how you felt last time you skipped breakfast? What do you think would help you feel good this morning?"

For kids who have the flexibility to eat a snack during school hours, you can also return to "Match Meals to Hunger Patterns" by packing a large snack for them to eat when they do feel hungry at school.

Scenario: Talking about how hungry or full your child feels.

While kids know their own hunger and fullness best, helping them find words to *describe* those feelings allows you to support them as the Food Leader by providing what they need and prepares them to do the same for themselves as they grow. This strategy builds on "Name and Normalize Sensations" but focuses on helping your child express what they feel during eating.

Talking About Your Child's Body Concerns

It can be heartbreaking to hear your child question their body, especially if you've had similar worries yourself. But these moments aren't about having the perfect response, they're about connection.

Scenario: Your child worries they are too big or too small or compares themselves to someone else's strength, speed, or abilities.

"Fixing" your child's feelings is a natural instinct, and you're not wrong to have it. But in these moments, what your child needs most isn't a quick reassurance—it's your Calm and Steady Presence and willingness to listen. By slowing down, you can help them feel truly seen and supported. Try the following strategy.

Strategy: Validate, Don't Dismiss

When your child shares worries about their body, it's natural to want to reassure them right away. After all, you *do* think they're perfect! But saying "You're perfect!" or "Don't think that!" can accidentally shut down the conversation and send the message that you don't understand what they're feeling, or it's not okay to feel the way they do. Instead, take a breath and validate what you're hearing, which opens the door for reflection and helps your child learn that all feelings—even the hard ones—are safe to talk about with you. You can say:

> "Sometimes it can be confusing when we notice our body is different from someone else's. I'm really glad you told me what you're feeling."

Once your child feels heard and understood, you can gently help them zoom out. The goal isn't to convince them that their body is "just right," but to emphasize that bodies come in all shapes, sizes, and abilities, and that difference is both normal and good. To do this, use the following strategy.

Strategy: Celebrate Differences

After you've created space for your child's feelings, you can gently widen the lens to emphasize that bodies are meant to be diverse. Talk about how people come in all shapes, sizes, colors, and abilities and that everyBODY has its own way of moving, growing, and changing. This will be most effective when you are already communicating these messages through your 3 Ms. Hearing this message from someone they trust who loves them unconditionally—you!—helps your child internalize that their worth isn't tied to size, shape, appearance, or ability.

"Bodies change and grow at their own pace, and yours is doing just what it's meant to."

When a child worries that their body is too large, many parents instinctively respond, "You're not fat; you're beautiful!" But this implies that large bodies *aren't* beautiful. And if your child *does* have a large body, this response can also dismiss their lived reality. Another statement parents sometimes use is "You're not fat; you *have* fat," similar to how the child has fingers and elbows. But unlike individual body parts, body *size* is part of our identities, just like race and neurotype. Instead of separating a child from the word "fat," we can help them understand that it is not an insult and that all bodies deserve respect, belonging, and care.

Lastly, we can teach our kids about how these feelings are rooted in an oppressive system, always in Developmentally Attuned ways.

Strategy: Call Out Oppression in an Age-Appropriate Way

Kids are quick to notice unfairness, and that's a powerful tool for helping them understand body oppression. When you name the injustice behind body ideals, you show your child that these ideas come from larger systems, not their or anyone else's individual worth. And when you do this over time, it helps them grow into compassionate, critical thinkers who question harmful messages instead of internalizing them. Here's what you can say about size oppression at each age:

Preschoolers (3–5 Years)

"Some bodies are big, some are small, and all bodies are good."
"When someone says mean things about a body, that's not kind or fair."

Early Elementary (5–7 Years)

"Our family believes that everyone deserves to be treated kindly, no matter what their body looks like."

Late Elementary (8–10 Years)

"When someone is left out or teased because of how their body looks, that's called discrimination, and it's wrong."

Tweens (11–12 Years)

"You might hear people talk about 'getting healthy' when they mean 'getting thinner'. Let's talk about what 'health' really means."

Teens (13+ Years)

"Anti-fat bias and unrealistic body standards are a kind of oppression. They hurt people and stop them from getting the support they need."

Talking About Other People's Bodies

This is a challenging topic, even for adults. On one hand, ideally comments about body size would be neutral descriptors, just like tall and short. But given the world we live in, words like "fat" can still feel hurtful, depending on who's hearing it.

> **Scenario:** Your child makes a comment about someone else's body.

Just like we teach kids about consent when it comes to touching someone else's body (and anyone else touching theirs), we can extend this principle to how we talk about bodies.

Strategy: Words About Bodies Need Consent Too

Everyone has the right to decide how others talk about their body. Even if your child means no harm, describing someone else's body can land as hurtful. Help your child understand that we can't always know how a word feels to someone else, so it's best to let that person decide. You can emphasize that curiosity about bodies is okay, but those comments belong in private conversations with you. Try saying,

"That person gets to decide how people talk about their body, just like you do about yours."

Bringing It Home

Talking about bodies with your child isn't about getting every word right. Every time you meet your child's concerns or curiosity with care and curiosity of your own, you're helping them see that bodies aren't projects to fix or reflections of our worth. They are a unique, valuable part of our identities.

By taking the time to have thoughtful conversations about bodies and grounding yourself in your Family Core Values, you show your child what it means to treat bodies with kindness and respect. And if you struggle to truly believe that your own body is good and worthy, of course this will be challenging at first. But just like talking about food, the more you practice, the more natural it will feel to talk about bodies with kindness and respect. Over time, your language supports your child's Body Trust, Self-Regulation, and Belonging and Identity and listen to their own body's needs for life.

One Simple Step: Modeling Body Trust

Practice saying what you feel in (or about) your own body out loud and without judgment, like "My stomach's starting to growl, I think it's time for lunch!" or "That stretch was just what I needed." This Models how to notice and care for your body's signals and shows your child that listening to their body is normal and important.

Your Food Positivity Practice
Finding the Right Words

17

Navigating Food Exploration (Making Food Fun for All Ages + Stages)

My son refuses to try anything new, and I'm running out of ideas. If I ask him to just taste it, he shuts down. If I leave it on his plate, he ignores it completely. I've tried making it fun, cutting veggies into shapes, offering dips, and even turning it into a game, but nothing seems to work. Sometimes I wonder if I should just stop offering new foods altogether because it feels like a battle every time. I want him to feel curious and confident with food, not pressured or scared, but I don't know how to get us there.

—Melissa

BY NOW, YOU understand why food exploration matters—how curiosity builds trust, why pressure backfires, and that giving kids time and space to explore at their own pace helps them feel safe and confident. And you've seen how Playful Exploration that's Experience-Based + Joyful nurtures Body Trust, encourages critical thinking, and builds real-life skills that reach far beyond the table.

Now, it's time to get practical. In this chapter, we'll walk through what food exploration can actually look like for kids of different ages and stages. You'll find easy, everyday ideas that slip right into your routine, no fancy prep, no long to-do list, just simple ways to spark curiosity and build confidence around food.

Each strategy ties back to the Food Positivity Framework and the Learning Foundations by keeping experiences Developmentally Attuned, Body Positive, Experience-Based + Joyful, and Inclusive. These aren't tricks to "get kids to eat." They're invitations for kids to discover, connect, and grow with food in ways that feel safe and fun.

What Does Food Exploration Look Like in Action?

At its heart, it's hands-on, low-pressure, open-ended play that helps kids feel more comfortable and curious around food. Exploration looks different for every child and can be tailored to age, development, interest, goals, and even location.

You can think of it a little like the Montessori method, where kids are offered purposeful tools, or the Reggio Emilia approach, where kids follow open-ended invitations. We follow the Kid Food Explorers *Explore-to-Grow Compass*™ a flexible, protective framework that blends the best of both weaving Food Positive learning into everyday life. It offers direction without pressure, honors each child's unique pace, and uses food as a playful, everyday medium for curiosity, confidence, connection, and capability.

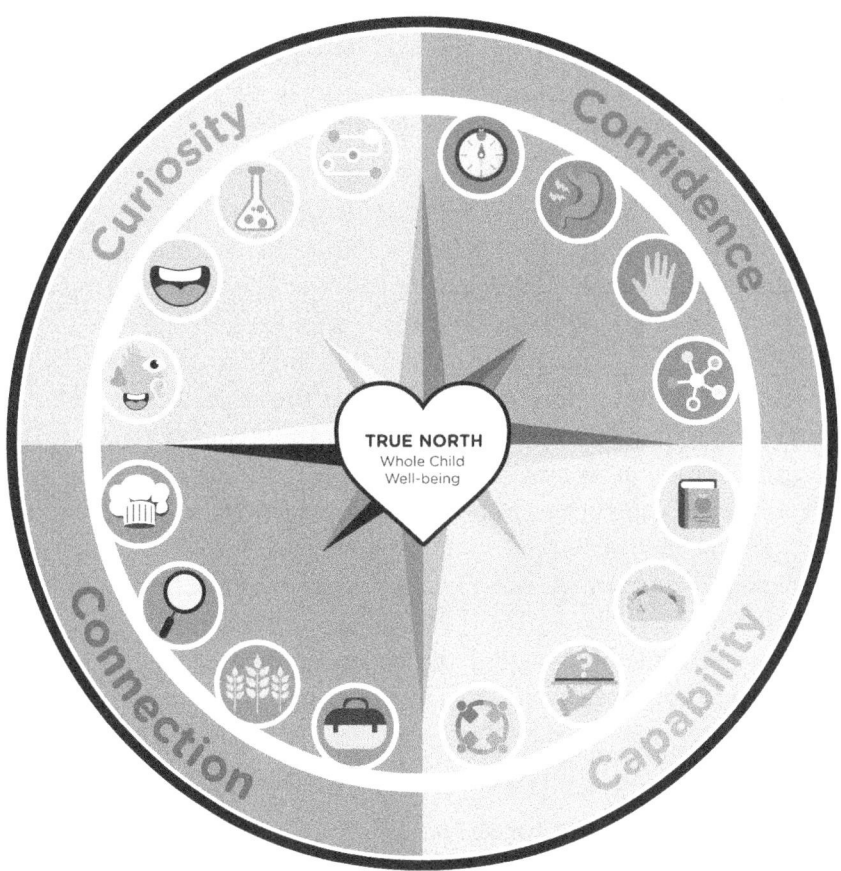

Centered on your Family Core Values, the Kid Food Explorers approach helps nurture Whole-Child well-being one small, meaningful moment at a time. Sometimes that looks like carefully set up experiences, such as comparing broccoli prepared three ways. Other times, it's completely child-led, like sniffing every spice in the cupboard just because it's fun. Both matter.

Food exploration is *not* a sneaky way to "get" kids to "just try one bite." Kids can sense when exploration is actually a hidden test or has an agenda, and that pressure can make them shut down. There's no tricking, no "gotcha" moments, and no clapping *only* when they finally taste.

> *The Explore-to-Grow Compass™* doesn't measure progress by what a child eats; it's measured by sparking curiosity, building confidence, creating connection, and developing capability.

Every squish, sniff, stack, and question counts as learning. A child spreading with a knife, building a "snacktivity" castle, or making up a story about tomato fairies in the garden, is all exploring. These small, playful moments matter more than any one single bite.

Food exploration doesn't just happen at the table. Reading a book about vegetables, learning the ABCs with fruit, going to a pumpkin patch, watching a cooking show, and even putting googly eyes on a melon that sits on your countertop until it's ready to be sliced – these all count. With the *Explore to Grow Compass™*, food learning can happen anywhere: in art, history, science, story time, and everywhere in between.

Always remember Playful Exploration works only when kids feel safe and respected. That means honoring their preferences, following their cues, and making sure their basic Growing Needs are supported.

The Language of Exploration

Before we get into the "what if my child. . ." scenarios, let's pause for a moment and talk about the *how*. The words you use during food exploration matter just as much as the activity itself. Your language sets the tone. It's the difference between an invitation that sparks curiosity and a comment that shuts it down.

Food exploration language should spark curiosity, affirm your child's Autonomy, and keep things open-ended. Instead of praising or pressuring, you're simply noticing alongside them. Instead of saying, "Good job for trying it!" you might say, "That texture is gritty, isn't it?" Instead of "Just try it," you might ask, "What do you notice about how it smells?"

When you shift from directing to wondering, food exploration becomes safe and playful and mealtimes become less stressful. It tells your child: *You get to decide* and *your experience matters*.

Some quick questions you can lean on in almost any exploration moment:

- "What does it remind you of?"
- "What does your body say about that?"
- "Want to see what happens if we. . .?"
- "Can you describe it using your senses?"
- "Is there anything about it that surprised you?"

These kinds of questions work across ages, whether your child is learning to flip pancakes, comparing different apple varieties, or pretending that the butternut squash you just bought is their newest babydoll.

Strategies That Always Apply to Food Exploration

Just like there are phrases that work almost anywhere, there are strategies you can lean on every time food exploration comes up. These practices can guide you no matter the age, stage, or setting.

Mindset Shifts: How You Show Up

Let Them Lead   Kids learn best when they're the explorers, not the audience. If your child wants to poke, sniff, name, or even walk away, that's part of it. You're following their pace, not your plan.

Celebrate the Process, Not the Outcome   It's easy to cheer when a child finally takes a bite, but bites aren't the only kind of progress. Exploration is about all the steps along the way: noticing the smell, swirling the spoon, stacking the crackers, or laughing at the funny shape of a carrot. When you name and celebrate those moments, your child learns that curiosity and comfort matter more than "performing" for approval. That's what builds real trust and confidence.

Less Is More   You don't have to fill every silence or coach every move. Sometimes the best support is saying less and noticing more.

A quiet smile, a nod, or a simple "I see you exploring" can be more powerful than explaining. Often, doing a little less and just being present, relaxed, and available makes the experience feel safer and more playful. This is Co-Regulation in action.

Trust That It's Enough   Even 10 seconds of curiosity is progress. You're planting seeds. Small explorations today become confidence tomorrow.

Language Tools: How You Talk

Invite, Don't Instruct   Exploration feels better when it's an invitation. "Want to smell it?" or "Want to touch its scaly skin? It feels like a snake to me!" This protects your child's sense of Autonomy.

Stay Curious Together   You don't need to be the expert; you just need to be curious alongside them. Try simple open-ended questions like:

- "What do you notice?"
- "How does that feel in your hands?"
- "I wonder what will happen if we mash this?"

Use Neutral, Descriptive Language   Skip labels like "healthy" or "junk." Instead, describe what you see, smell, hear, feel, or taste: "This one feels silky" or "That tastes tangy." Words shape meaning, build vocabulary, and neutral words build Body Trust.

Ground Lessons in Real Food, Not Abstract Nutrients   Skip teaching nutrients in isolation, like "Carrots help you see in the dark." Keep learning grounded in real, lived experience before building toward abstract concepts. Kids understand food best when it's connected to something they can see, touch, taste, and feel because that's how their bodies and brains make meaning.

Practical Supports: How You Make It Work

Honor Preferences   Not every child likes the same food, and not every exploration ends in a bite. Honor your child's taste bud and texture preferences.

Celebrate All Kinds of Interactions   Each child has different interests and likes to explore in their own way. Offering tools like tongs, gloves, or even just inviting kids to observe and decide if they want to join in can be supportive. If you know your child loves dinosaurs or unicorns, find a way to make their interests part of the process because even pretending counts. Exploration is inclusion.

Belonging Starts with Feeling Welcome   Make space for every child's food, body, and traditions to be seen and celebrated. All foods are good foods; all bodies are good bodies.

Build Skills That Last a Lifetime   Food exploration is confidence in action. From whisking and measuring to planning and creating, kids aren't just making food; they're developing capability, creativity, and problem-solving skills that grow with them.

One important thing to remember is that kids are *learning eaters*. Just like they're learning readers, writers, and problem-solvers, food exploration is how they learn. By approaching food learning from a growth mindset perspective and creating space for curiosity, mistakes, and trying again, we shift the focus from "getting it right" to growing through the experience. That's what helps kids build confidence and resilience, not just around food but in all areas of life.

Food Exploration for Responsive Scenarios

You can use food exploration for real-life in-the-moment situations to reduce pressure, build trust, and support your child's Autonomy and curiosity. These moments can happen during meals, snacks, or food-related conversations when you might not have even planned to teach them anything, but a powerful opportunity for learning presents itself. Responsive exploration helps kids build comfort with new or unfamiliar foods, supports their sensory needs, and creates safety without the pressure to eat.

> **Scenario:** Mealtime is stressful or there's a power struggle between you and your child.

It's easy to slip into control battles at the table. But if every meal feels like a showdown, everyone's guard goes up. Food exploration invites curiosity back in and creates connection instead of conflict.

Strategy: Make Mealtimes Playful, Not Pressured

You can reduce your child's anxiety and create a safe learning space by playing pretend or giving food silly names. Try:

"Let's pretend we're lions tonight and eat like a lion. ROAR!!! I wonder what I want to eat first?!?"

"I'm having wiggly worm noodles (pasta), clown mustaches (red peppers), and dragon eggs (grapes) for dinner tonight! Do you want some crunchy pirate coins (cucumbers) on your plate?"

Strategy: Create a Reset Ritual

Transitioning from conflict to connection helps re-regulate both you and your child. Try this activity:

Invite everyone to do a 10-second "shake it off" wiggle dance. Then try again with a deep breath and a reset: *"We were feeling stuck, let's try again. No one has to eat anything, but let's just sit and be together."*

> **Scenario:** Your child says, "That's gross!" or makes a face.

You just served dinner. Your child side-eyes one of the foods or calls it "gross," and now the whole mealtime vibe feels tense. This is an opportunity to support your child's learning without shame or control.

Strategy: Notice and Transition

This is a four-part strategy. First name what you notice to help diffuse tension and model curiosity.

1. "You made a face, looks like something surprised you. Wanna tell me what you noticed?" Or "Hmm, sounds like you weren't expecting that smell. That's okay, let's explore together."
2. Then, with "Use Positive Language" from Chapter 15: "We use kind words to talk about food."
3. Take it a step further with a kid-friendly way to encourage respect at the table with the phrase: "Don't "yuck" my yum."
4. Then follow up with curiosity: "What didn't you like about it? Was it the texture or the flavor?"

This kind of language builds food literacy and communication skills. Over time, kids learn to say "It's a little too spicy for me" or "It feels squishy in my mouth" instead of rejecting unfamiliar foods outright.

Strategy: Encourage Growth Mindset Language

Giving kids the agency and language to express their preferences without a hard "no" is a powerful way to leave an open invitation that they might like it one day. It also shifts the focus to process over outcome. Encourage kids to say:

I'm still exploring it.
Taste buds can change…
I'm still getting to know it.
I'm still learning about this food.
My taste buds are still deciding.
My taste buds are still learning.
I'm learning about this flavor.
Maybe I'll like it another time.
My tongue needs more tries.
It's not my favorite right now.

Strategy: Normalize Dislike as Part of Exploration

This strategy reinforces that not liking something is okay and the goal isn't *liking*; it's *learning*.

"This food is not my favorite, I'm still exploring it."

> **Scenario:** Your child wants only familiar foods.

You serve up a balanced plate with a variety of foods and hope they'll at least try the veggie. But before you can blink, they've cleared the pasta and asked for more while the broccoli remains untouched. Also check out "Gentle Exposure" and "Modeling Variety Yourself" from Chapter 15.

Strategy: Offer Food in Multiple Varieties or Forms for Discovery

Seeing the same food in different varieties or prepared in different ways can bridge curiosity toward new items. Try this activity:

Include different varieties of the same food (like two types of apples) on the table and narrate getting curious about them. Invite your child to become a food explorer and use their senses to investigate carrots that are raw, steamed, and roasted with cinnamon sugar.

Strategy: Pair Familiar Foods with Playful Exploration

Keeps mealtimes positive and encourages curiosity around other foods without taking away the comfort of the preferred food.

Strategy: Practice "No Big Reaction" Parenting

Kids learn what matters to us by what we react to. If we over-focus on the bread, we send a signal that it's powerful and that other foods are a battle. You don't have to say anything to practice this strategy. In fact, it's better if you don't!

> **Scenario:** Your child says, "I'm not hungry" (even though they haven't eaten much).

They say, "I'm not hungry," again or maybe they just push the food around It's easy to spiral: *What if they wake up starving? Are they manipulating me?* But this moment is *not* a test, it's a trust-building opportunity to honor their body cues.

Strategy: Keep Meals Low-Stakes but Engaging (Note, This May Feel Like Pressure to Some)

Being around food still builds confidence even if they don't eat. Inviting little curiosity invitations can feel helpful for some kids. Try saying:

> "Want to be a food explorer and see what this feels like in your fingers? You don't have to eat it, just curious what you notice."
> "Want to help stir the soup or sort the crackers by shape while we chat at the table?"

Try this activity: Invite them to help pass food, smell something new, or compare shapes ("Do you think the cucumber is longer than the spoon?"). These micro-moments count!

> **Scenario:** Your child surprises you by trying something new.

You weren't expecting it, but they poked it with a fork, licked it, or maybe even tasted it. However it looked, this is a *huge* moment. But what happens next matters just as much as the taste itself, because how you respond shapes whether food exploration feels safe and empowering to your child. . .or loaded with pressure and performance. Try the following.

Strategy: Celebrate Without Pressure

Using encouraging language supports your child's confidence without adding expectations for next time you serve this food.

"You tried it, what did you notice?"
"I love how curious you were to explore that!"

Strategy: Avoid Labeling the Moment

Praising your child as "a good eater" can backfire by turning food into a performance. Instead, you can say:

"Looks like you're listening to your body."
"You're learning about what you like."

Food Exploration for Active Learning Moments

Food exploration isn't just for stressful moments or responsive scenarios. That's the beauty of it; it can happen anywhere, anytime! In fact, if you do have a Learning Eater, using food as a playful teaching tool outside of mealtimes is powerful. You may remember in Part II when we talked about the benefits of food exposures. This is how you make them meaningful and pressure-free. When kids explore food through play, stories, culture, science, or art, they're not just learning about food; they're learning about the world. These intentional moments help expand their diet variety, build food literacy, and connect kids to their culture and Family Core Values, all while nurturing Food Positivity.

Bonus Handout via the QR Code: Food Exploration for Active Learning Moments

Bringing Food Exploration to Life

You've got the mindset, so now let's make it real. Food exploration isn't about *doing* more; it's about *noticing* more. Here are simple ideas to use at any age, with any food, in any setting.

Infancy (0–12 Months): Build comfort with textures, smells, and the joy of exploration. Every messy moment builds comfort and brain connections.

- Place a few soft foods (mashed avocado, banana, cooked carrot) on their tray for squishing, smearing, and touching.
- Offer two foods in contrasting colors (orange sweet potato, green pea) and let them look and reach.
- Narrate, "This smells sweet!" or "You found the slippery one!"

Toddlers (1–3 Years): Build familiarity and trust through repetition and freedom to say "no." Narrate their discoveries like "You noticed the orange one feels soft!"

- Stack berries or banana slices on skewers (or straws).
- Sing about foods ("The Tomato Grows on a Vine") or make up silly verses.
- Let them stir, pour, or sprinkle in small tasks.

Preschool (3–5 Years): Turn food exploration into imaginative, sensory play. At this age, play = learning and curiosity is your best teacher. Books can make new foods feel familiar and guessing games like which foods will float or sink in water is fun.

- Go on a "rainbow food hunt" in the fridge or store.
- Explore the sounds foods make when chopped, stirred, or shaken.
- Stamp with bell pepper tops or okra pods in mustard or paint.

Bonus Handout via the QR Code: Children's Books That Support Food Exploration

Early Elementary (5–7 Years): Build confidence through small responsibilities and real-world participation. The goal isn't trying new foods; it's helping them learn about their own taste buds and texture preferences.

- Try one food prepared three ways (raw, roasted, baked, blended, jellied, dried, etc.).
- Ask them to read simple instructions or ingredient lists aloud.

- Keep a "Food Explorer Journal" to track their discoveries with draw, describe, or rate by senses (not "like/don't like" and why).

Late Elementary (8–10 Years): Deepen curiosity; start questioning messages about food and bodies. Start connecting exploration to culture, identity, and media awareness.

- Choose a family tradition or friend's culture to explore through food.
- Read labels for ingredients or country of origin and learn more about how they are grown in that country.
- Germinate seeds and plant them in a garden.

Tweens (10–12 Years): Build agency and connection while learning about food together and talking about it.

- Let them plan a dinner within a budget.
- Discuss food myths together and look for real info.
- Encourage them to make snacks or meals for family or friends.

Troubleshooting Common Stuck Points

- **"When they still won't taste":** Don't worry, you're still making progress! Stick with touch, smell, and food exposures outside of mealtimes. You can also help your child learn about their flavor and texture preferences to find foods and preparation methods that align with those preferences.
- **Worries about food waste:** Let them serve themselves, always start with offering less and let them add more.
- **Stressing about the mess:** Contain it with mats, towels, damp cloths, or one "messy" night a week.
- **Siblings or comparisons:** Say: "EveryBODY is different. EveryBODY learns at their own pace."
- **Big or small appetites:** Start with structure around meals and snacks and minimize food pressures.
- **Neurodivergent needs:** Safe foods, predictable plating, sensory supports, and attuning to your individual child's needs.
- **History of pressure or trauma:** Repair aloud and go slow. Try "I pushed bites before, I'm sorry. Let's start tuning-in together."

Bringing It Home

It's easy to feel inspired and overwhelmed at the same time. Remember, you don't have to do everything. In fact, the most meaningful change often comes from doing less, from slowing down and letting curiosity guide you (and your kiddo).

When curiosity replaces control, meals stop feeling like battles and start becoming opportunities for connection. Whether you're clipping herbs in your garden, comparing the same food prepared in different ways, or reading a food-themed story before snack time, every small moment counts.

It's not about adding more to your day with big experiments or planning themed dinners (unless you want to!) These are moments that already show up in your everyday life, where you can invite your child to explore and follow their lead. Because when we foster Playful Exploration, confidence naturally follows. And that supports Food Positivity for life.

One Simple Step: Say Less, Notice More

Pick a food, new or familiar, and simply explore it together without any goal of eating. Let your child take the lead while you practice saying less, noticing more, and celebrating curiosity instead of bites. *You're not teaching about food, you're learning about your child.*

Your Food Positivity Practice

Moments of Wonder

18

How to Handle Food and Body Talk from Others (and Support Your Child Too)

Last year at Thanksgiving, my mom pinched my son's side and said, "He's getting a little chubby, time to cut back on all those snacks!" She smiled like it was a heartfelt joke, but he didn't eat much for the rest of the gathering. My first instinct was to just laugh it off, because that's how I'd always handled those kinds of comments from her myself. But I wanted to say something about it this time. I realized I'd heard that same tone my whole childhood, and I don't want my son to have the same experience.

—Morgan

PLENTY OF CARING adults in your child's world still operate from diet-culture values. And while we hope to see lasting change in dismantling those beliefs, for now it's an unfortunate reality. Others may label foods, comment on bodies, or pressure kids to eat a certain way, all in the name of "health." Sometimes these messages come from a place of love or concern, like an older relative repeating what they were taught or a teacher trying to encourage "healthy choices." And usually, they're so normalized that others don't even realize the harm these messages cause.

As parents, we can't control what others believe or say, but we *can* decide how we respond. Every time you calmly address these

271

moments—whether you're setting a boundary with another adult or helping your child make sense of what they heard—you're reinforcing your Family Core Values through the 3 Ms. You're showing your child that food and body talk don't have to be unsafe or shameful. They can be opportunities for connection, clarity, and care.

This chapter will help you do both: advocate for your child's safety *and* guide them through confusing or harmful messages when they arise. You'll see how to respond in real time to the people sharing harmful messages, all while strengthening your child's Food Positivity Protective Shield so they can grow up feeling confident in their body and grounded in their own beliefs, even when the world around them isn't there yet.

Boundaries: Your Tool for Protecting Your Child (and Yourself)

Boundaries are an important part of supportive leadership. In Chapter 12, we explored how the Division of Responsibility helps you and your child maintain boundaries with *each other* to keep mealtimes supportive and rooted in trust. Now, we'll take that same concept beyond your family table and into the wider world to help you set boundaries that protect both your child and your own mental health.

Boundaries are not punishments or power plays. They're clear decisions about *how we will respond* to protect our child—and within the Food Positivity approach, it can help to take another look at Chapter 5 because what you are specifically protecting are your child's Growing Needs and Skills. You also get to protect the hard work you're doing on yourself to stop viewing your food choices or bodies as reflections of our worth—*your* Felt Safety, Body Trust and Autonomy, and your Family Core Values.

Quick gut-check: If the goal is to "make them change," that's not a boundary, that's control. But if the goal is to "keep myself and my child safe and living in alignment with our Family Core Values," that's a boundary.

Build Your Boundaries with A.N.C.H.O.R.

When harmful messages or actions show up in your child's world, you may struggle to figure out exactly how to step in. And as we'll see in the next chapter, sometimes you actually won't need to. As your child's Food Positivity Protective Shield grows stronger, they'll be able to recognize harmful messages for what they are, put them aside, and take actions that support their own self-care.

But when your child is young and still building their Protective Shield, establishing boundaries with other people in their world to protect their ability to develop the Life Skill of Food Positivity is an important part of your role as their steady, attuned leader.

If you grew up in a home that valued control and obedience, we know that speaking up can feel very uncomfortable. You might even find yourself needing to set boundaries with the very people who once expected your obedience. This will stir up lots of old emotions and uncertainty, but that's okay. Take a breath. Your discomfort is a sign that you're doing something brave and different: protecting your child while breaking cycles that began long before you.

Since most of us didn't grow up with anyone Modeling how to create calm, respectful boundaries, we created the **A.N.C.H.O.R.** tool to help you navigate challenging situations while staying *anchored* in your Family Core Values.

Each step helps you advocate for both yourself and your child as well as reflect internally on your actions and reactions to ensure they're in line with your Family Core Values. When you hold boundaries with your Calm and Steady Presence, it shows your child that their needs matter more than anything to you. And over time, it teaches them how to set their own boundaries and stay grounded in their values as they grow.

Notice how some of the steps in **A.N.C.H.O.R.** are *internal* reflections and decisions you make, while others are *external* things you communicate to others. Let's see how it works.

> **Scenario:** You're at a family meal. Another adult says to your child, "You need to take three more bites before dessert" or "That's too much bread, have some salad first."

A—Assess the situation (internal): First, pause and notice what's happening and whether it could be genuinely harmful to your child. Notice not just what the other person said but how it's affecting your child—and you. Ask yourself:

- *What's actually happening right now? How is my child responding? Are they handling the comment just fine, or do I need to step in?*
- *What's my own emotional state? Am I calm enough to take action right now?*

This quick check helps you figure out when to step in and when it's okay to wait or ignore the comment because your child's Protective Shield is already doing its job. But if your Attunement tells you your child feels uneasy or unsafe, that's your cue to act. Pausing to reflect helps you take actions aligned with your true goal—to keep your child safe and supported—instead of reacting from heightened emotions.

N—Name what matters (internal): If you've determined that taking action is the right move, take another moment to clarify what's most important in this situation, the needs and values you seek to protect. Ask yourself:

- *What's at stake here for my child? How might this compromise their Growing Needs and Skills?*
- *Which of our Family Core Values is being crossed or dismissed?*
- *What do I want my child to take away from how I handle this moment?*

Naming these things to yourself helps again helps you stay *anchored* in what matters most to you and your child, so your external actions reflect the safety and care you want your child to feel.

C—Communicate clearly (external): Next, communicate your boundary. When the person you're talking to is someone who truly trusts and respects you, a **light response** should be all that's necessary. This actually isn't even a boundary yet, just a request that someone who respects you will likely honor. Note how these statements are rooted in your Calm and Steady Presence. This might sound like:

"Oh actually, we let [your child] decide what and how much to eat from whatever is part of the meal. Thanks for understanding."

If the situation continues, that's a sign that the other person isn't ready to honor your approach or respect your values that guide it. So you can move to a **firmer response** such as:

"I know you care about [your child] eating well. We're following an approach that keeps food relaxed and positive, so I'd really appreciate you no longer making those comments."

Here, you can take actions to support your child, like moving to sitting between your child and the person commenting, or redirecting the conversation. But if the behavior continues, it's time for a **hard response**, the actual boundary you establish to keep your child safe, such as:

"I'm sorry, but if you keep pressuring [your child] to eat, we're going to need to wrap up for now and visit again another time."

H—Hold the line (external): Boundaries lose meaning when they're only words. This is the step where you follow through, again with your Calm and Steady Presence. Do what you said you'd do, whether that's ending the conversation or removing yourself and your child from the situation.

Remember that holding the line still isn't about control, even though others may interpret your actions that way. You have the agency to take actions that support yourself and your child—period. Following through on your boundary with confidence shows your child their safety comes first and reminds others that your boundaries aren't up for debate. Avoid a heated confrontation if you can. Just like in your parenting, you can respond with empathy while still holding firm, Modeling to your child that boundaries and kindness can coexist.

O—Open repair (external): Once the moment has passed, take time to reconnect, with both your child and, when possible, the other adult involved. Repair doesn't mean apologizing for holding a boundary. It's about restoring trust and understanding after tense moments.

With your child: Focus on reassurance and safety. They may still feel uneasy or confused about what happened, especially if someone they care about was involved. A quick, calm follow-up helps them process what they saw and reminds them that you're their steady base. You might say:

> "I stepped in because it's my job to keep you feeling safe. You can always count on me for that."

With the other adult: Circle back later, when everyone's calm. Remember that your goal isn't to debate your values, it's to clarify your boundary and preserve the relationship if possible. You might say:

> "I value our relationship, and I'm hoping we can keep food talk positive and pressure-free next time. Are there any questions about my approach I can answer for you?"

Repair doesn't erase what happened. It strengthens connection by showing that supportive boundaries and relationships can coexist. This step teaches your child that you're always acting from your Family Core Values, even in difficult situations.

R—Reflect and reset (internal): Once the situation has passed, take another moment to reflect privately. This isn't about replaying the interaction or judging how you handled it—it's about learning from it. Ask yourself:

- *Did my response keep my child feeling safe and supported?*
- *What worked well, and what felt hard?*
- *Is this a relationship I can continue safely, or do I need more distance?*

You might also consider whether a **proactive boundary** could help prevent similar situations in the future. For example, you could clarify expectations before a meal ("Let's keep food talk positive today") or adjust where your child sits next time.

Each time you pause to reflect on a moment when you implemented a boundary and what happened as a result, you strengthen your own Calm and Steady Presence and supportive leadership—and your child's trust that you'll support their needs, no matter what happens.

A.N.C.H.O.R. in Action

Now let's see how A.N.C.H.O.R. works in real life. In the examples ahead, you'll see that we've focused on the external steps (Communicate Clearly, Hold the Line, and Open Repair), because those are the actions you'll take in the moment. The Food Positivity Practice at the end of this chapter will help you with the inner work (Assess, Name, Reflect), which are just as important and can take some getting used to, especially if you're not used to prioritizing your own needs.

> **Scenario:** Another adult keeps talking about their diet or weight loss in front of your child.

When another adult begins talking about their diet or weight loss around your child, it can be tricky to know how to respond, especially if this is someone you care about. Remember, your goal isn't to convince them that dieting doesn't work—they have the autonomy to make their own choices, too. It's to protect your child's and model calm, confident leadership.

If the relationship feels trusting and respectful, this strategy can help you Communicate Clearly with a **light response**:

Strategy: Lead with Shared Care

When another adult begins discussing their diet or weight loss in front of your child, remind yourself that most people who talk about dieting are acting from care—they believe they're modeling "health." Beginning from a place of shared care helps you stay anchored in Body Respect and your Calm and Steady Presence. It also shows your child that standing up for *your* values doesn't mean conflict; it means communicating from kindness and conviction.

Light Response (gentle redirect): *"Oh, we really don't want to give [your child] any ideas about dieting. Kids are impressionable and I imagine you don't want them getting any ideas about dieting either. Tell me about your weekend instead!"*

If the comments continue, you can acknowledge the person's likely good intentions while firmly protecting your child's boundary.

Firm Response (restate values + clarify impact): *"I know you care about your health, but we really try to avoid weight and diet talk around [your child]. Preventing disordered eating is really important to us, and we want them to feel confident in their body."*

And if it continues, it's time to introduce your boundary to protect your child, always with your Calm and Steady Presence.

Hard Response (boundary): *"I'm just not comfortable with [your child] continuing to hear about dieting and weight loss talk from you. If you plan to continue talking about it, we're going to have to head out."*

And to follow through: *"My child's safety has to come first. We're going to (head outside, leave early, etc.)."*

Later, perhaps in the car or another calm moment, Open Repair with your child:

> "That was a lot of talk about [adult's] diet! Do you have any questions for me? Remember, in our family we don't judge bodies or food and we can always eat enough to feel full. You're doing a great job listening to your body."

If you can, follow up privately with the adult later, Open Repair, again using "Lead with Shared Care"

With the other adult (privately): *"I know that conversation probably felt awkward. We're trying to protect [your child] from weight and diet talk so they can build a healthy relationship with their body. I know you also want what's best for them. I don't need you to understand my reasons, I just need you to trust that my actions are about keeping my child safe."*

If the other adult is open to it, you can always share more resources on the approach you're using, but you don't actually *need* them to understand so long as they can agree to respect your boundaries.

Scenario: Another adult makes a harmful comment about your child's body.

When someone comments on your child's body—whether it's meant as a joke, a compliment, or something else—it can quietly chip away at their Body Trust. While outright criticisms are clearly harmful, even well-intentioned compliments about size can send the message that their worth depends on staying the same, leaving them to wonder if they'll still be valued if their body changes.

This is one of those times when you don't need to start gently. You can jump right in and Communicate Clearly with a firm response, using the following strategy.

Strategy: Name the Value, Not the Violation

Naming the violation is still important sometimes, but emphasizing what *you* stand for rather than what the other person did wrong can help you stay grounded in your Calm and Steady Presence and keep the situation from escalating. This approach teaches your child that protecting their dignity doesn't have to require heated conversations. It can simply be about standing up for Family Core Values like safety, agency, and individuality.

Firm Response (state values + clarify impact): *"We really prioritize helping [your child] feel safe and confident in their body. Comments about appearance can make that harder, so we'd appreciate it if you avoid them altogether. Thanks for understanding."*

This is often the point where adults you're setting boundaries with may interpret your actions as control or disobedience—especially if *they* grew up in environments that valued compliance over communication. Stay rooted in your Calm and Steady Presence. You don't need to defend your choice or win them over. Simply follow through and give yourself permission to decide what kind of contact or communication feels best to you moving forward. They get to have their feelings and values, and you get to have yours. The following strategy can help you Hold the Line.

Strategy: Protect Your Family's Peace

Sometimes protecting your child's safety means recognizing that another relationship isn't safe to continue as is. Repeated harm through body comments, diet talk, or shaming—especially when you've established boundaries to keep this talk away from your child—shows that the other person just isn't able to respect your values. You can create distance calmly and clearly, limiting contact or changing the setting so your child isn't exposed to ongoing harm. You might say:

> "I care about our relationship, but I have to protect [your child] from messages that could contribute to body shame or disordered eating. I've made several requests about this that you haven't honored, so I'll be limiting our time together until I can be sure you will respect my boundaries."

This is a firm boundary, and you have every right to hold to it, regardless of how the other person feels about it. And "Protect Your Family's Peace" doesn't mean closing off your heart. It means leading with care while keeping your family safe.

After your child hears harmful comments about their body from someone else, use your Attunement to figure out how the comments may be affecting them and Open Repair with a comment like:

> "That comment about your body wasn't okay. I'm sorry you had to hear that. Your body is strong and good just as it is, and I'll always speak up if someone says otherwise. If you have any feelings about that comment you want to share, I'm here to listen."

Scenario: A staff member at your child's school or daycare comments on your child's food or tells them they need to eat it in a certain order.

In Chapter 20, we'll take a closer look at how schools can teach kids about food in a more Developmentally Attuned way. But comments about your child's lunch or snacks aren't part of the formal curriculum, and they're often an area where you can step in right away.

When addressing these situations, approach staff calmly and respectfully, knowing they've likely done things this way for a long time. These comments are usually well-intentioned efforts to "encourage healthy eating," but they may not align with your Family Core Values, and it's okay to say so. The following is a helpful strategy here.

Strategy: Curiosity Before Correction

This approach honors the other person's expertise while allowing you to stand in your own. Starting with genuine curiosity keeps the exchange collaborative instead of defensive and models your Calm and Steady Presence. Once you've listened and understood their perspective, you can share your own Core Family Values and clarify why it's important to you that staff members not speak to your child in a way that may compromise their Growing Needs, without needing to prove who's right.

If the comment came from your child's teacher, you may already have a direct line of communication with that person. But more often, teachers are pretty busy with other tasks during student meals, and it's a parent volunteer, paraprofessional, or other school staff member who helps supervise lunch. In those cases, you can take your concerns to the school's administrative staff. You can start the conversation with:

Light Response (gentle outreach): *"I wanted to check in about something [your child] mentioned. Someone at lunch told them they needed to eat their sandwich before they could eat the cookies I packed. I know everyone wants what's best for the kids, so could you tell me more about the school's approach to mealtimes?"*

You may find that the administrative staff was unaware of these kinds of comments coming from other adults during mealtimes and they're happy to have a conversation with the volunteer or staff member about letting your child choose "whether" and "how much" right away.

But if you discover that the school doesn't approach feeding kids the way you do, you can use "Lead with Shared Care" to continue the conversation:

Firm Response (state values + clarify impact): *"I really appreciate how much everyone here cares about the kids' well-being. We're working with [your child] to help them trust their own hunger and fullness cues, so I'd like to request that staff and volunteers let them choose how to eat their food on their own."*

You might also consider sharing this bonus handout with the staff:

Bonus Handout via the QR Code: Food Positivity Mealtime Message

And to Open Repair with your child, focus first on reassurance through your Calm and Steady Presence:

With your child: *"You didn't do anything wrong when that grown-up told you how to eat your lunch. In our family, you get to decide what to eat and when. I talked to the school so they understand this too."*

Doing so helps restore your child's Felt Safety and Body Trust and reminds them that even when others get it wrong, you'll step in to ensure that other adults will support their needs as well—Modeling a skill that will certainly serve them well as adults.

> **Scenario:** Someone has told your child something about food or bodies that doesn't align with Food Positivity.

This is one of the biggest concerns we hear from parents. In the next chapter, you'll learn that while these kinds of messages aren't disappearing anytime soon, the work you're doing to strengthen your child's Food Positivity Protective Shield will prepare them to navigate such moments with confidence. But when children are young, they're especially impressionable. Comments about "healthy" and "unhealthy" foods—or about calories, sugar, bodies, etc.—can easily take root.

How you Open Repair with your child in these moments is a powerful opportunity to reinforce your Family Core Values through the 3 Ms. You can adapt "Call Out Oppression in an Age-Appropriate Way" from Chapter 16 here, as well as use the following strategy.

Strategy: "Some People Think That"

Before you focus on correcting the message itself, try helping your child understand (in a Developmentally Attuned way) that some people have different beliefs about food and bodies than your family. They may have been told things that led to negative thoughts about certain foods or body types, but *you* know in *your* family that all foods and all bodies are good. By calmly explaining this and even empathizing with the person who made the statement—that while their belief is likely unhelpful and can cause stress, it's something they were taught themselves—you help your child see that those messages aren't facts. they're opinions shaped by the world around us. This opens the door to critical thinking and keeps the conversation rooted in your Family Core Values. Try statements like the following:

Preschoolers (3–5 Years)

"Some folks were told sugar is bad, but we know desserts can be part of our delicious meals!"

Early Elementary (5–7 Years)

"People don't always agree about what's 'healthy'. Our family believes health is about doing what feels right for your body."

Late Elementary (8–10 Years)

"Sometimes people talk about calories or sugar because they've learned to worry about it. We focus more on listening to our bodies, eating all different kinds of foods, and enjoying them!"

Tweens (11–12 Years)

"Many people believe there's one 'right' body, but our family celebrates how bodies change and grow."

Teens (13+ Years)

"Diet culture convinces people that they need to control their food or bodies to be accepted. I want to help you feel confident that you get to make your own choices about what you like to eat, and your body is just right for you."

You can also encourage critical thinking in these moments (something we'll take an even closer look at in the next chapter) by using this strategy, which builds on "Lead with Curiosity" from Chapter 16.

Strategy: Support Body Trust with Curiosity

When your child shares something they've heard about food or bodies, take a curious approach. Give them space to share what they noticed and how it felt before you offer your perspective. This shows them that food and body talk aren't dangerous topics or conversations you'll shut down right away with correction. Your child is safe to explore these confusing messages with you. Staying rooted in your Calm and Steady Presence helps your child stay connected to their own inner cues too, supporting Body Trust and strengthening their Food Positivity Protective Shield. Try:

> "What did you think when you heard that?" "How did that make you feel about your food (or your body)?"

And if the person who made the comment was another adult and you have the opportunity to Communicate Clearly them, try the following responses rooted in "Lead with Shared Care" and "Curiosity Before Correction":

Light Response (gentle outreach): *"I wanted to touch base about something [your child] mentioned. They said someone told them [specific comment]. Could you share a bit more about what was said?"*

If the adult confirms the comment or seems unaware of its impact, use warmth and structure together. Here, you validate their intent while clarifying the effect on your child.

Firm Response (state values + clarify impact): *"I understand the goal might have been to teach about health, but we're helping [your child] learn that all foods and bodies are good. When they hear that a food or body is 'bad', it can make them feel anxious or ashamed."*

And: *"Thank you for understanding how important this is to us. I appreciate your support in keeping that message consistent."*

But if the comments continue, Hold the Line with a boundary that protects your child's safety:

Hard Response (boundary): *"I need to be clear that moral or negative language isn't something I want [your child] exposed to. I'll need to [no longer visit with you, opt them out of these lessons, etc.] if this continues."*

Bringing It Home

Setting boundaries and responding to your child when others talk about food and bodies in harmful ways is hard. You might feel uncertain or stumble over your words at first and then replay the moment later wishing you'd said something different. That's okay. These moments aren't about saying everything perfectly. With practice, you'll find your footing. Your child may not remember every word, but they'll remember how your actions made them feel and that you were their steady guide, always anchored in your Family Core Values.

And whenever you Communicate Clearly, you show your child that it's safe to talk about hard things and that their body is worth protecting. You Model what it looks like to stand up for your values with confidence and empathy. Each conversation helps them build the language and courage to advocate for themselves someday. And that memory becomes a lasting reminder that they can trust your care—and, in time, their own voice too.

One Simple Step: Practice Boundaries Out Loud

Choose one boundary you've been hesitant to voice—a diet comment, a body remark, a food rule—and practice your response in a mirror or with a partner. Saying it out loud helps your body learn what calm authority feels like, so when the real moment comes, your words will flow from steadiness, not stress.

Your Food Positivity Practice

The Inner Work of Boundaries

PART

V

Raising the Next Generation

19

A Systemic Change for Transforming the Food and Body Environment

We didn't talk much about calories or weight when I was growing up, but the vibe was definitely that making healthy choices was the responsible thing to do. In high school, I read an article about "clean eating," and the idea of sticking to only the "right" foods felt empowering, almost like a badge of honor. I read labels, skipped foods my friends ate, and was really proud of my willpower. But by college, trying to eat "clean" was controlling my life. Figuring out a more balanced relationship with food took years, and I often wished I'd had more support to realize what was happening sooner.

—Tori

WE SO OFTEN hear from parents that while they're trying their absolute best to raise their kids with a positive relationship with food and their bodies, there are just so many outside influences rooted in diet culture, it feels like it's impossible to protect them completely.

It can feel like all the work you're doing to protect your child could be undone by something they'll encounter in the world that you have no control over.

And while in many scenarios (with teachers and relatives) you can absolutely stand up for your child via the scripts we shared in the previous chapter, the truth is diet culture *is* all around us. We can keep our homes safe through positive language and unconditional support for our kids' unique needs, but the more independent they become, the more they will encounter messages shaped by diet culture outside of your home.

But *your* child will have something you likely didn't have: the Food Positivity Protective Shield you've built through the 3 Ms and your Family Core Values.

So when body ideals, a careless comment, or another harmful message comes their way, it won't sink in as deeply as it may have for you. Instead of going straight to their heart, they'll have the tools to pause and ask themselves, *"Is that really true? "The world has lots of ideas about food and bodies, but I don't have to believe all of them."*

The World Outside Your Home

Children don't just face one kind of outside influence—they grow up surrounded by overlapping layers that all carry messages about food and bodies. Some of these layers are close, like teachers, friends, and extended family. Others are more distant, like cultural norms, media, and public policy, yet they still shape the environment your child moves through every day. Together, these layers interact to form the broader ecosystem your child is learning in.

That can feel daunting, especially if you remember how deeply these same influences shaped you growing up. But because of the work you're doing in your home, your child isn't entering these systems defenselessly.

When we understand how these layers work, the picture becomes less overwhelming and more empowering. You can start to see more clearly where the pressures come from and how your home environment anchors your child as they filter those messages. To see just how these layers work, let's take a closer look at the Ecosystem of Food and Body Learning that we introduced to you in Chapter 7—how each layer shapes your child's world and how your support helps them navigate it.

Rooted in Research, Expanded for Reality

We've already explored the first layer of our Ecosystem of Food and Body Learning—your child's home environment, aka the microsystem. Now, we're taking a look at the outer layers of the Ecosystem, again adapted from Bronfenbrenner's Ecological Systems Theory. We've updated it with Neo-ecological insights to reflect today's digital world where kids learn from home, school, and screen. We've also woven in perspectives from Intersectionality and Culturally Responsive Teaching, because not all kids receive the same messages about food and bodies. Racism, anti-fat bias, ableism, and classism show up in everyday places from lunchrooms, grocery aisles, to doctor visits. When we see what's shaping our kids, we can start to shift it.

The Ecosystem of Food and Body Learning

Your unique child is at the center of their environment, with your 3 Ms shaping their earliest and most influential beliefs about food and bodies. In Chapter 10, we explored how moving away from negative values like obedience, conformity, and healthism—and leaning into supportive, positive values—creates a strong foundation for Food Positivity at home.

Now let's take a look at the broader ecosystem your child is growing up in and how each layer—from close relationships to large cultural forces—shapes their learning about food and bodies and how your actions through the 3 Ms create protective thoughts your child can lean on when they encounter diet culture messages.

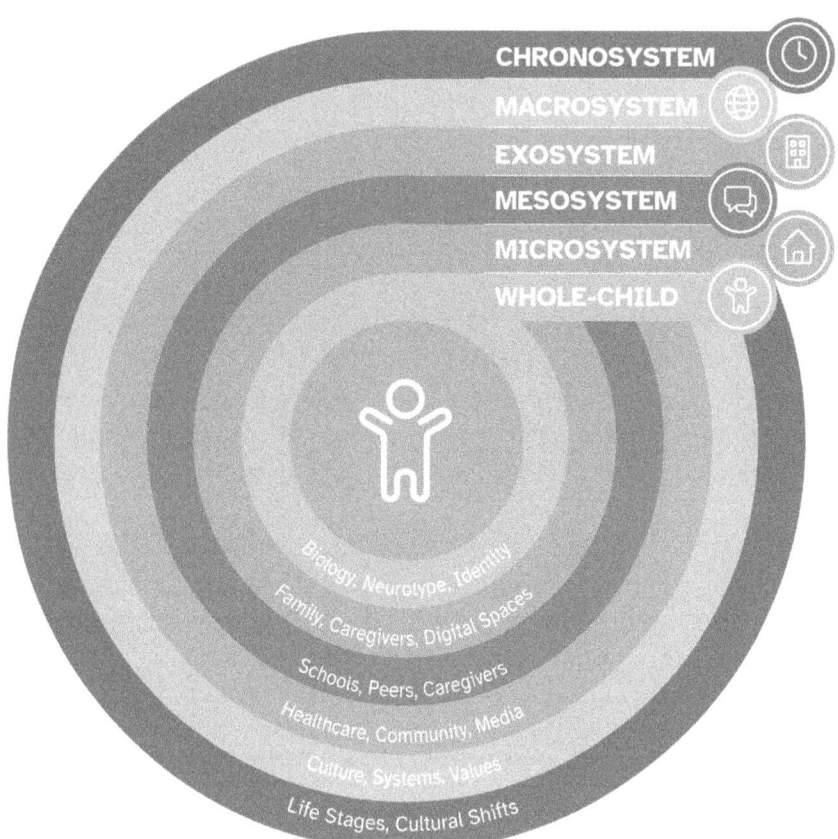

The Whole-Child

Every child brings their own biology, temperament, lived experiences, neurotype, sensory needs, and cultural background and identity into their learning. That means what works for one child might feel overwhelming, confusing, or even harmful to another. Supporting them well starts with knowing them well.

Microsystem: Home, Close Relationships, and Online Spaces

This is where your influence is strongest, through daily routines, conversations, and connections. It's how you respond when they say, "I'm full," or "I feel fat." It's the tone you use when offering dessert. It's your own relationship with food and your body, showing up moment by moment. It also includes the people who feel like part of your child's everyday life, like the cousin who's over after school, the neighbor who eats dinner with you twice a week, or the friend who spends whole weekends at your house. Their words and behaviors shape the atmosphere, too. And then there are digital spaces your child visits like a cooking show on YouTube, a lesson on an educational app, or even a video game, that may plant ideas about which foods are "healthy" or what bodies are more accepted. These virtual moments may seem small, but they're part of the learning environment, too.

Mesosystem: Schools, Caregivers, and Social Circles

This layer includes all the places and people your child interacts with on a regular basis. From teachers and coaches to babysitters, grandparents, and friends, it's where different messages might collide or compete. Sometimes, these overlapping environments show up in digital spaces, too. A friend's comment about "junk food" at lunch might show up again in a shared video or a teacher's message about acceptable snacks might be reinforced in a school app.

Why it matters: Kids may get praised for finishing their lunch at school but encouraged to stop eating at home. They might hear comments about "processed" snacks at a friend's house or see different rules for siblings. These inconsistencies can create confusion or shame. You can't control every environment, or every message that pops up on a screen, but you can help your child process those experiences and offer clarity through your consistent presence and Family Core Values.

Mesosystem: Filtering Outside Messages		
Outside Message (Negative Values)	Parent's Past Action (Core Values in Action)	Child's Protective Shield Thought/Action
A peer has been talking about how they want to lose 10 pounds (*conformity, perfectionism*).	Parents have consistently celebrated body diversity and talked about how people thrive in many different shapes and sizes (*individuality*).	*"Bodies aren't supposed to all look the same. I don't need to diet, my body is good as it is."*

(*continued*)

(*continued*)

Mesosystem: Filtering Outside Messages		
Outside Message (Negative Values)	Parent's Past Action (Core Values in Action)	Child's Protective Shield Thought/Action
A school health lesson teaches about "good" and "bad" foods (*perfectionism, control*).	Parents have consistently shown that food is not a moral issue and that vegetables, cookies, and pasta all have a place at the table (*positive leadership, joy, and wonder*).	*"I know food isn't about being good or bad. I can enjoy all kinds of foods."*

Exosystem: Community, Media, and Institutional Influence

This layer includes systems your child may not interact with directly but that still shape their everyday experiences. Think about the media you're playing in the background, healthcare visits, school food policy, advertisements, grocery store layouts, or your own stress from work or finances. Even subtle things like algorithm-driven ads on a tablet or a school lunch app's red-yellow-green food codes can quietly deliver messages about food and bodies that influence how your child feels about eating.

Why it matters: These systems influence how food is accessed, how bodies are treated, and what's seen as "normal." For example, a lack of affordable fresh food in your neighborhood or a doctor's casual comment about BMI can shape food and body narratives in powerful ways.

Exosystem: Filtering Outside Messages		
Outside Message (Negative Values)	Parent's Past Action (Core Values in Action)	Child's Protective Shield Thought/Action
A commercial promotes a "healthy" product with no added "junk" (*healthism, perfection*).	Parents have normalized flexibility in eating, making room for desserts, traditions, and spontaneity (*connection, joy, and wonder*).	*"That ad is just trying to make people afraid of food. I don't need to be scared. Eating is joyful and all kinds of foods can fit."*

Exosystem: Filtering Outside Messages		
Outside Message (Negative Values)	Parent's Past Action (Core Values in Action)	Child's Protective Shield Thought/Action
A doctor comments that the child's BMI indicates "overweight" and parents should monitor their food intake (*healthism*, *control*).	Parents have emphasized that bodies grow in different ways and focused on how the child feels, plays, and learns, not the scale (*individuality*).	*"I shouldn't have to go hungry. My body is unique and worthy, not defined by a number."*

Macrosystem: Culture, Power, and Ideologies

This is the big picture, the beliefs and structures that shape our society. It includes diet culture, racism, anti-fat bias, ableism, healthism, and moralized food narratives. These messages shape how children learn to measure worth, value, and belonging. Digital culture is part of this, too. What goes viral, who gets praised, and which foods or bodies are centered or mocked online all reinforce bigger societal patterns.

Why it matters: Not all kids experience the same level of safety or acceptance when it comes to their bodies or cultural foodways. Children in larger bodies, disabled kids, Black and brown kids, and children from immigrant families often face bias earlier and more intensely. That's why creating a food-positive, identity-affirming home is so powerful. Your Family Core Values become the strong foundation and everyday language your child can lean on as they learn to navigate a culture that often gets it wrong.

Macrosystem: Filtering Outside Messages		
Outside Message (Negative Values)	Parent's Past Action (Core Values in Action)	Child's Protective Shield Thought/Action
Media trends present thin, white, able-bodied individuals as the standard of beauty and success (*conformity, achievement*).	Parents have exposed their child to diverse role models, celebrating stories and accomplishments not tied to appearance (*individuality, joy, and wonder*).	*"When media focuses on one kind of body, that's harmful. Everyone deserves to see themselves represented with dignity."*
News stories warn about the "obesity" epidemic, linking processed food land lack of willpower to body size (*healthism, self-sacrifice, conformity*).	Parents have emphasized dignity and respect for all body sizes, discussed the SDoH and shared stories of role models in diverse bodies (*well-being, individuality*).	*"Health is more complex than that. People deserve access to quality food and supportive care without being pressured to change their size."*

Chronosystem: Time and Life Transitions

This layer recognizes that beliefs and behaviors change over time. Puberty. Divorce. Moving. Social media. Global events. Even your own healing journey. All of these transitions shape how kids (and adults) understand food and bodies across their lifespan. As children move into the tween stage, new experiences like getting their first phone, joining a class messaging app, or watching short-form video content can spark new questions, comparisons, and sometimes new beliefs.

Why it matters: Big shifts like starting school, hitting puberty, or scrolling TikTok can bring up new questions and challenges. This layer reminds us that learning isn't linear, and we always have the opportunity to grow, revisit, and repair along the way.

Chronosystem: Filtering Outside Messages		
Outside Message (Negative Values)	Parent's Past Action (Core Values in Action)	Child's Protective Shield Thought/Action
After joining social media, the child's algorithm starts showing them content about food restriction and body ideals (*obedience, healthism, self-sacrifice*).	Parents have consistently talked about media messages critically and modeled a wide variety of body-affirming, food-positive voices (*agency, individuality*).	*"I don't need to follow content like that. I can choose to scroll past, block, or seek out creators who make me feel good."*
Starting college, the child notices many peers skip meals or brag about not having time to eat (*self-sacrifice, achievement*).	Parents have modeled that nourishment and rest matter, even during busy or stressful times (*well-being, connection*).	*"Even if others don't make time to eat, I know fueling my body helps me feel and do my best."*

Critical Thinking: Your Child's Inner Filter

Each of the Protective Shield examples you just read is really about one thing: critical thinking. This is precisely what we've been working toward all along in helping your child develop their Food Positivity Protective Shield. Critical thinking means pausing to notice a message, considering it against their own experience (your Family Core Values and the 3 Ms), and deciding whether it aligns with what they know to be true. That ability to stop and reflect is one of the most powerful skills you can give your child, and its benefits extend far beyond food and body conversations.

> "To raise a critical thinker means giving our kids opportunities to discover what they know intimately and their barriers to understanding."
>
> —Julie Bogart, *Raising Critical Thinkers*

If you didn't grow up with the parenting style and values we've encouraged throughout this book, chances are you had fewer opportunities to practice these critical thinking skills. That may explain why questioning diet culture's harmful messages feels harder for you now. And that's *not* your fault. Both authoritarian and permissive parenting styles make developing these skills more challenging—authoritarian with its emphasis on obedience and conformity, and permissive with the lack of guidance kids need to strengthen critical thinking skills.

But responsive parenting—paired with a strong foundation of your Family Core Values—helps critical thinking thrive. When children feel both supported and guided, they have the freedom to question, reflect, and practice making choices within safe boundaries.

Fostering critical thinking in your child also shifts your role as a parent, because instead of trying to control every setting or shield every influence, you become the guide. You help your child build their *own* filter.

Over time, our kids learn that they don't have to accept every message at face value; they can pause, question, and choose what aligns with who they are and what they believe: *their* values. That's how they grow into kids and eventually adults, who navigate the many layers of influence they'll encounter as they grow.

Spotting Diet Culture in Everyday Media

One of the first places your child will practice critical thinking is in how they process the media they consume. Many parents worry about their children's screen time and media consumption, and for good reason. Excessive or unsupervised screen use has been linked to a range of problems in children, from attention to anxiety. Research also shows that media exposure can play a role in the development of eating disorders, as children who are still building their critical thinking skills are more likely to absorb harmful messages about food and bodies at face value.

It's natural to want to protect your child from messages that could undermine their confidence or shape harmful beliefs. And you can, especially in the younger years when their brains are still "under construction," with supportive boundaries relating to their screen and social media use.

The challenge is that diet culture is so deeply woven into our world that it often slips into content that is still incredibly valuable for its humor, creativity, or positive life lessons. Think of Blippi identifying "healthy" options in a grocery store or Bluey's parents expressing a desire to change their bodies.

Moments like these remind us that even well-intentioned children's media often reflects society's narrow views of food and bodies. Rather than shielding kids from every questionable message, your most powerful move is to keep the conversation open—naming what you notice, asking questions, and practicing media literacy together.

Media Literacy: Helping Kids Understand What They Hear

Media literacy is critical thinking applied to media. It's noticing when an image might be AI-generated, recognizing marketing and advertising tricks, and realizing that a social feed is carefully filtered to look "perfect." It's the ability to see how these messages shape ideas about health, beauty, success, and belonging—and to notice when they're designed to make us feel inadequate or sell us something. And it's the skill of asking, "What's the message here? Who does it serve? And how does it make me feel?"

By naming what you notice and helping your child think critically, you give them the tools to navigate media with confidence and stay rooted in your Family's Core Values:

- "I wonder why Blippi said, 'An apple a day keeps the doctor away.' I had an apple yesterday, and I still went to see my doctor about my allergies! What do you think?"
- "How do you think Peppa Pig's dad feels when they joke about his big tummy? I don't think I would like someone to talk about my body like that."
- "Have you noticed that a few of the movies we watched recently had a greedy villain with a large body? Do you think someone's body size actually tells us if they're greedy?"

As kids grow, you can widen the lens: ask what an influencer gains by promoting a product, why larger-bodied characters are often cast as sidekicks rather than leads, or how an ad uses fear to sell a supposed "fix." The goal isn't to lecture but to spark curiosity and show that it's normal to question what we see.

- "Do you think that influencer really looks like that, or are they using a filter?"
- "That YouTuber keeps talking about those snacks. Do you think they really eat them every day, or are they being paid to talk about them?"

Over time, these conversations build your child's ability to think critically, stay rooted in your Family's Core Values, and notice harmful cultural norms about food and bodies. And as they age and gain exposure to additional media messages, they'll be increasingly able to pause, ask who benefits, and decide for themselves whether a message aligns with what they know to be true about worth, health, and belonging.

Quick Takeaways to Encourage Critical Thinking

- **Consider the message:** Teach kids to recognize when someone is making a claim about food, bodies, or health instead of just absorbing it passively.
- **Ask who benefits:** Encourage them to ask, "Who benefits from sharing this message?"
- **Compare with your values:** Help them ask, "Does this fit with what we believe about food and bodies?"
- **Practice together:** Model out loud how you question and evaluate messages you're both hearing.
- **Keep it low-pressure:** The goal is curiosity, not getting the conversation exactly right. Small, consistent conversations add up.

The Media You Consume

Of course, it's helpful to consider the media *you're* consuming as well. We're living in a peak era of nutrition and wellness misinformation. The teen magazines we once poured over have been replaced by "fitspo" and "what I eat in a day" content that glorify restriction and reinforce narrow body ideals.

When it comes to feeding your kids, you're likely hearing fear-based wellness claims from influencers and online voices. They blame sugar, dyes, or preservatives for the "state of children's health," even though there's little evidence to back those claims. These messages hit home because caring for our kids is our deepest instinct. Of course we want to protect them. And they play on the anxiety parents likely already feel about the state of the world and the *true* risks to children—things like poverty, lack of quality healthcare and education, and violence—with fear-based advice that offers us something actionable and concrete to do, even if the advice is shaky at best.

And even when feeding advice comes from nutrition professionals, an unfortunate reality is that disordered eating is even *more* common among those who enter nutrition careers than in the general population. Those disordered beliefs can slip into the resources they create. On social media, this is often where we see the Food Talk Traps we covered in Chapter 9 and misapplications of DOR in Chapter 12: control-oriented tactics repackaged in a shiny, family-friendly wrapper.

By practicing critical thinking around what *we* consume and grounding our choices in science, trusted expert voices, and the kind of support we know our unique children need, we strengthen our ability to nurture Food Positivity in our kids.

EXPERT INSIGHT: The Business of Making Parents Feel Bad

Megan McNamee MPH, RDN of @feedinglittles, co-author of *Feeding Littles Lunches* (Rodale, 2024)

Do you know why scrolling online feels so overwhelming as a parent right now? Because creators are fighting for your attention and they have to say polarizing, judgmental, or ridiculous things to get it.

They likely make you feel like crap about yourself because odds are, you've done one of those things. You start consuming this kind of content, reading the comments, and trying to learn

(continued)

(*continued*)

more to help yourself feel better, which causes that platform's algorithm to keep pushing that type of content to you. Suddenly it feels like "everyone" knows how to parent better than you do, you're "messing it all up," and if you don't do it all X way, you're getting it wrong. But that's simply not true.

What's worse, a lot of the information is objectively incorrect. Anyone can build an online platform and teach online. But it still makes us feel terrible about how we parent because we keep seeing examples of what we're doing wrong.

Just know that parenting content on social media has become more stressful than ever, and it's not because you're doing something wrong.

Advocating for a Better World

Make no mistake: While we can prepare our children to navigate diet culture with resilience, that doesn't make it okay that our culture continues to elevate narrow body ideals and sustain structural inequities that make true well-being harder for many families.

It can feel overwhelming to recognize how deeply diet culture and body stigma are woven into the world your child is growing up in. But that doesn't mean you're powerless. Speaking up plants seeds of change, whether by advocating for more inclusive health lessons in your child's school district, calling your political representatives about funding for critical health programs in your community, or sharing a resource about eating disorder prevention with another parent.

You may also choose to support organizations and movements working to shift cultural norms: nonprofits promoting body diversity in media, groups advocating for quality food education in schools, or campaigns fighting weight-based bullying. These efforts matter because oppressive systems rely on silence and complicity to hold their ground. And every act of speaking up not only challenges an oppressive culture; it models to your child that your Family Core Values extend far beyond your home.

"I swore never to be silent whenever and wherever human beings endure suffering and humiliation. We must always take sides. Neutrality helps the oppressor, never the victim."

—Elie Wiesel, Nobel Peace Prize acceptance speech, 1986

And remember, none of this has to happen all at once. Advocacy doesn't mean fighting every battle; it can simply look like small, steady choices that align with your values and fit within your capacity. What matters most is that you use the influence you *do* have, however limited it may feel, to make the world around your child just a little more supportive, inclusive, and Food Positive.

Advocacy in Action

Here are practical ways you can push back against diet culture and weight stigma, at a level that works for you:

- **In your child's school district:** Create trusting partnerships with school staff members and share the importance of supporting kids while eating with positive language and not using pressuring feeding tactics. Volunteer to create bulletin boards or other displays that emphasize body diversity and celebrate cultural foods.
- **On kids' teams and activities:** Encourage coaches and activity leaders to keep the focus on skill-building, teamwork, and fun rather than body size, calories, or "working off" food. Speak up when language about weight or restriction comes up, and suggest positive alternatives that celebrate effort, growth, and enjoyment.
- **In your community:** Speak up when you hear harmful conversations about weight and eating patterns, especially as they relate to children. Share books, podcasts, or articles that align with Food Positivity with friends, parenting groups, or faith communities. Sometimes a resource sparks reflection better than a debate.

(continued)

(*continued*)

- **On a larger scale:** Support organizations working for body-inclusive, anti-diet change, whether through volunteering, donations, signing petitions, or amplifying their messages online.

Bringing It Home

Even if you're doing everything "right," your child still lives in a world that often sends harmful messages about food and bodies. You can't protect them from every comment, ad, or lesson, but you can give them a strong foundation. You can create a home where they feel safe, valued, and like they belong.

Every moment of connection, every pause before commenting, every time you sit down to eat together without pressure or shame, every time you speak out about something unjust, those moments stack up. They create the kind of foundation your child can stand on when the world gets noisy.

"Even if your home is diet-culture free, your child still lives in a culture that isn't. That's why how we talk—and how we help them talk—matters so much."

You're not just shaping how your child eats. You're shaping how they see themselves and their role in the world. And that's one of the most powerful things you'll ever do.

One Simple Step

The next time you notice a message your child hears that is rooted in diet culture—on a show, in a school assignment, or even in a casual conversation—pause and name it. Ask a question like, "What do you think about that?" You don't need a perfect answer. Just starting the conversation will strengthen their Protective Shield.

Your Food Positivity Practice
Diet Culture Detective: *Spotting Hidden Messages*

20

Partnering with Schools to Redefine Food Education

Last month, my son's class did a lesson on "go, slow, whoa" foods. He came home and told me that fried chicken and macaroni were "whoa" foods and that eating them would make him unhealthy and cause too much fat on his body. But those are the foods my dad often makes on Sundays. We always look forward to it. The next weekend, he barely touched his plate, saying he was trying to be healthy. His school is so wonderful; I never expected it to be the place where he learned to be embarrassed about the foods our family loves.

—Jordan

BESIDES HOME, FEW places influence kids more than school—and that includes their formal lessons about food and bodies. Understanding how current lessons are shaped by well-meaning but biased views of health and nutrition and how they can be harmful is the first step toward advocating for education that truly supports their well-being.

If you were a kid in the '90s, you probably remember the iconic PSA campaign *The More You Know*, complete with the rainbow shooting star. That assumption is exactly what drives many of the nutrition programs in schools today. They're designed to educate and empower.

And on the surface, it makes sense. Most of us were taught that learning the "right" health facts would lead to better choices. But, just like we unpacked in Chapter 9, *how* we teach kids about food matters just as much as *what* we teach.

Maybe your child is learning about MyPlate at school, sorting foods into "stoplight" categories of green, yellow, and red, or saying things like "sugar is bad." Maybe someone got in trouble for bringing candy in their lunchbox, or you got a letter about approved "healthy" snacks you're allowed to send. Your child is watching, learning, and making meaning from it all.

If something about this doesn't sit well with you, you're not imagining it. Many school-based nutrition lessons are developmentally mismatched. While well-intentioned, they're still rooted in diet culture and not aligned with how kids actually learn about food and bodies that we outlined in Chapter 8.

The problem certainly isn't individual teachers with diet culture-driven agendas. Teachers care deeply about their students and want the best for them. Many are required to follow district-approved materials that are designed to meet state standards, leaving them with little flexibility regarding the lessons they teach. The real issue is the broader culture of health messaging that shapes those guidelines and curricula and filters into classrooms.

Let's take a closer look at what's missing from most food education, why even well-intentioned lessons lead to confusion or harm, and what a better approach could look like: one that's rooted in the Food Positivity Learning Foundations and supports your child's whole well-being.

Why "Healthy Choices" Lessons Can Hurt More Than They Help

To be fair, some research suggests that certain school-based programs can change kids' short-term eating behaviors. Studies may show that kids who learn about "healthy" eating and beverage choices reach more often for fruits and vegetables in the cafeteria line or reduce their intake of sugary drinks. Sometimes, they even show small changes in weight outcomes across a semester or school year.

This can make it look like nutrition education in schools is a straightforward success story. But nearly all of this research overlooks the unintended consequences and lacks long-term follow-up. These studies don't check for whether kids leave the classroom with negative feelings about their food choices or bodies. They don't capture whether a well-meaning lesson on "healthy choices" leads to food anxieties. And unfortunately, there is evidence that health education can be one of the many triggers leading to an eating disorder.

This blind spot matters. As we have seen, children are impressionable, and when health lessons link certain foods or body types with a child's character or sense of making "good choices," the harm outweighs any small short-term nutritional gains.

Why It's Hard to See the Problem

Part of what makes these lessons so tricky is that they don't look harmful at first glance. In fact, they often look fun and perfectly suited for kids. These lessons use playful methods like songs, games, and sorting activities that seem perfectly designed for kids' at that age.

But here's the mismatch: the teaching *methods* (the how it's taught) are often spot-on, while the *content* (the what is taught) is often wrong.

True developmentally appropriate practice requires both pieces to line up:

1. **The right methods:** Approaches that match how kids think, process, and engage at that age/stage.
2. **The right content:** Information kids are actually ready to understand at that stage of development.

Truly attuned practice also pays attention to each child's unique pace of development and prioritizes cultural responsiveness. This is why so many parents feel uneasy but can't quite put their finger on why lessons feel off. The activities look engaging, but the underlying messages leave kids confused, anxious, or even ashamed.

Science vs. Nutrition Lessons

If you look at common science lessons and standards, it's taught step-by-step.

K–2: Students explore living things and basic body parts through concrete, hands-on lessons.

Grades 3–5: They learn about individual body systems (digestive, circulatory, skeletal, muscular), before gradually building toward more abstract ideas about how those systems interact.

Now, let's compare that to health-focused nutrition lessons:

K–2: Rather than learning through fun, hands-on food exploration, kids are often taught to sort foods into "healthy" and "unhealthy," with abstract claims about how food will help or harm their bodies, concepts they aren't ready to understand.

Grades 3–5: Just as science class is introducing organs and systems, nutrition lessons jump ahead to metabolism, "calories in versus calories out," and how sugar relates to diabetes.

The mismatch is striking: science builds slowly and developmentally, while health-focused nutrition lessons skip ahead, often relying on fear instead of curiosity. If nutrition followed the same developmental model as science, kids would actually leave with real, lasting understanding instead of shame and confusion.

Why School Nutrition Lessons Reflect a Bigger Systemic Problem

Most of the time, what kids learn about food and nutrition in school health classes doesn't come directly from their teachers. It comes from state or district-approved curricula shaped by national guidelines like the Health Education Curriculum Analysis Tool (HECAT). The problem is, when those guidelines are influenced by diet culture and healthism, the lessons that follow end up misaligned with what kids are ready to learn.

Take one real example: a Pre K–2 grade standard that asks kids to "demonstrate effective refusal skills to avoid unhealthy food choices and promote a healthy eating pattern." If that's the expectation, then a curriculum has to be designed to match it. So a teacher might receive a lesson plan with playful activities and worksheets all focused on identifying "healthy" versus "unhealthy" foods, and that's what they're expected to teach.

If the standards themselves aren't developmentally appropriate for five- to eight-year-olds, every lesson created from them will be off-base, too.

Instead of teaching about the bigger realities that shape health— like whether families can afford groceries, have safe places to play, or have access to healthcare—kids end up learning that their well-being depends on picking the "right" foods and avoiding the "wrong" ones. Their hidden takeaway? If their body changes or their health is poor, it's their fault.

Kids Aren't in Charge of Their Health

Even if we accepted diet culture's idea that health is all about personal choices, it still wouldn't make sense to teach kids from that perspective.

Children don't buy the groceries, cook the meals, or decide if they can play outside unsupervised even in a safe neighborhood. They can't sign themselves up for soccer, get to practice on their own, or book a doctor's appointment. And they certainly can't decide whether to get a flu shot.

Expecting kids to manage their health is like handing them car keys when their feet can't even reach the pedals. It just doesn't make sense.

Their only job right now is to be kids: learning, growing, and knowing they're cared for.

What Counts as Food and Nutrition Education

Not all food learning is the same, and it matters.

Nutrition education is the most common. It focuses on nutrients, health outcomes, and "healthy" eating from a Western lens. Lessons may include sorting foods into categories and labeling them like "sometimes" foods and "switcheroos," identifying added sugar and solid fats and relating weight status and poor health.

Food education is hands-on and experience-based with a focus on teaching about foods from farm to fork. Lessons may include learning about where food comes from, how it's grown, gardening, taste-testing, cooking, and how it connects to culture, family, and identity. It's meaningful concrete real-world learning, though it's often left out of formal curricula.

Food literacy is an even broader view of food learning that teaches real-life skills such as shopping, cooking, tuning into body cues, identifying personal food values, and questioning food marketing. It prepares kids to navigate food choices with confidence long after the MyPlate posters come down.

Where School Nutrition Lessons Go Wrong

You're likely spotting the patterns of disconnection between development and food and body education. And when these lessons happen in a school setting, kids who are often the most vulnerable—like kids in larger bodies, kids with feeding differences, kids whose cultural foods aren't represented, or families with limited food access—often feel ashamed, excluded, or that they don't belong. Classrooms are supposed to be places where kids grow, not just in reading and math but in curiosity, problem-solving, critical thinking, and social-emotional learning. But when food lessons miss the mark, they can actually work against those goals.

Let's take a closer look at some common themes in school food lessons and unpack why they often cause more harm than good.

It Teaches Kids to Feel Bad About the Food They Love

Kids hear food labels like "healthy versus unhealthy," "good versus bad," or even "fuel versus fun" foods and internalize them as judgments—not just about the food but about themselves. When a snack is labeled a "red light food" or "junk," a child may feel ashamed for eating it or, worse, for enjoying it.

This can be especially harmful when those foods are cultural staples, sensory-safe options, or what's most available at home. Framing them as a problem sends the message that some bodies, families, or cultures are less worthy.

> A child comes home upset with a note from the teacher saying their snack wasn't "healthy." The crackers their parent packed, one of the few foods they reliably eat, were called "unhealthy" in front of the whole class. What was once a safe food and space is now a source of shame.

It Ignores How Kids Actually Learn

As we explored in Chapter 8, young children are concrete thinkers. They need clear, tangible experiences, not abstract ideas like "heart health," "balanced diets," or "preventing disease." But many food lessons use these big-picture terms without context, hoping they'll motivate healthy habits.

When kids don't understand what they hear, they fill in the gaps with fear or misinformation. This developmental mismatch leads to confusion, fear, and often rigid or distorted beliefs about food.

> A child hears that "too much sugar causes diabetes." One day, their friend collapses on the playground. A teacher explains to the class that they had low blood sugar from diabetes. Now the child is confused and scared. They begin refusing all sweets, even a slice of birthday cake, afraid they'll get sick too.

It Tells Some Kids Their Food (and Their Family) Don't Belong

Food education often reflects a narrow worldview: Western, white, able-bodied, and middle-class. It promotes foods like quinoa, cauliflower, and berries as "healthy," while labeling many cultural staples, like white rice, potatoes, and plantains, as unhealthy or inferior.

These lessons also tend to ignore sensory needs, food insecurity, or different cultural practices. It implies only certain foods (and by extension, bodies and cultures) are acceptable. When kids don't see their foodways reflected or, worse, hear them criticized, they begin to internalize harmful messages about their identity, culture, and worth.

> During a MyPlate lesson, kids are asked to draw a "healthy plate." A child proudly draws arroz con pollo and tostones, their abuela's specialty. The teacher says, "That's okay, but next time try to limit fried foods and add a vegetable." The child erases their picture and starts asking why grandma "doesn't cook healthy."

It Centers Obedience, Not Safety, Body Trust, or Curiosity

Traditional food education often trains kids to follow rules—like eat more of this, less of that—rather than explore, question, or reflect. Behavior-based systems such as sticker charts for trying new foods, praise for clean plates, or being labeled a "good eater" train kids to seek approval from others instead of tuning into their own body cues. For kids who live in food-insecure homes, have sensory needs, or lack autonomy over what's served, these expectations can feel confusing or even impossible.

> A child is praised at school for always finishing her lunch. She starts asking at home, "Did I eat enough? Did I do a good job?" even when she's clearly full. Instead of trusting her body, she's now seeking approval.

It Teaches Kids to Fear Their Bodies and Judge Others

In some lessons, food isn't framed as nourishment; it's framed as a way to avoid weight gain or manage disease. Kids are told things like "You'd have to jump rope for five minutes to work off a piece of chocolate, but only one minute for an apple" or "High fat foods can narrow the arteries and make it hard for your heart to work. This can slow our bodies down." These scare tactics don't build health literacy; they build fear, shame, and body distrust.

Kids in larger bodies, kids with feeding differences, and kids from food-insecure homes are especially vulnerable to these messages. And because children repeat what they hear, this quickly turns into peer judgment and body policing.

> A child in a larger body brings a candy bar to aftercare, a rare treat. A classmate calls out, "That's why you're so fat. All you do is eat candy bars." This might've been the child's first candy bar in months and their only snack that day.

Pulling Back the Curtain

Now that we've looked closely at school food lessons, it's easier to see the bigger picture. On the surface, these lessons look different. Some show up as catchy songs about "good" and "bad" foods. Others have cute stories that frame choices as "sometimes" versus "everyday" foods. Some compare sugar grams or fat content in different snacks. But underneath, they share the same root problem: They rely on control. Instead of helping kids listen to their bodies, they teach kids to follow external rules.

So it's natural to wonder, if this isn't working, how should schools be teaching kids about food? Scaring, shaming, and excluding aren't effective, but surely kids need to learn something about food and health. And the truth is, schools are uniquely positioned to nurture food skills in the same way they nurture music, art, or computer science.

Imagine if food lessons weren't about rules, labels, or vague warnings. Imagine if they started with curiosity, connection, and care. Instead of memorizing nutrients and "bad" foods, kids might explore why rice looks different across cultures, plant a seed and watch it sprout, or notice how eating a snack helps them focus better in math. When food learning is grounded in safety, trust, and joyful, hands-on exploration, kids don't just learn facts; they build lifelong confidence and critical thinking.

This is where the Food Positivity Learning Foundations come in. They give us a new perspective, one that aligns what kids are ready to learn with how schools actually teach. They shift food education away

As we like to say, it's not about teaching less; it's about teaching better.

from fear and control and toward the conditions kids need to thrive: developmentally attuned lessons, inclusive stories, and experiences that spark curiosity and connection.

Bringing the Learning Foundations to Life Through Food Exploration in Schools

The same Learning Foundations don't just guide families at home; they can transform how schools approach food education. When lessons are Developmentally Attuned, Body Positive, Experience-Based + Joyful, and Inclusive, food stops being about fear and control and instead supports children's growth, confidence, and sense of belonging.

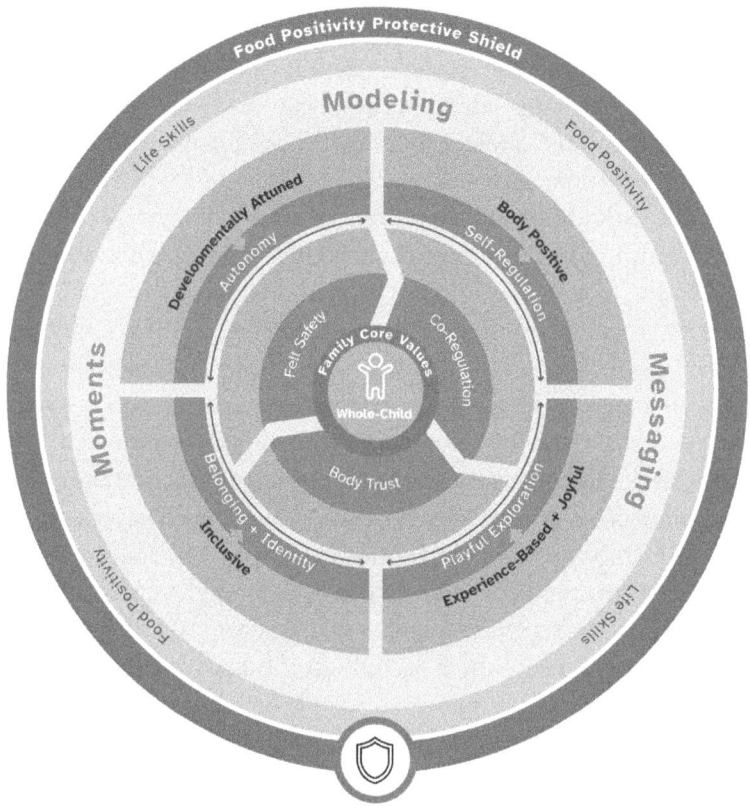

Food exploration is how the Learning Foundations come to life in schools.

It's not an "extra" activity to squeeze into the day; it's a natural, hands-on approach that enriches what schools already do and can meet learning standards. Just like science labs, art projects, or music rehearsals, food exploration is cross-curricular, a bridge between learning and life. It supports science when students sprout seeds, math when they graph taste-test results, literacy when they write food poems, and social-emotional learning (SEL) when they share family food stories and traditions.

By weaving food exploration into existing subjects, schools make learning developmentally meaningful, culturally responsive, and joyfully integrated.

This isn't just about nutrition; it's about using food as a lens for Whole-Child learning, connecting curiosity, culture, and community through everyday experiences.

Developmentally Attuned in Schools

Kids make sense of food the same way they learn science or math: start concrete, and then build layer by layer. Younger children might explore colors, textures, or where foods come from. Older students can connect food to body systems or try simple experiments. Teens may unpack how marketing and social media shape what they believe. When lessons grow this way, kids feel grounded. They think, *This makes sense. I can learn this.*

Food Exploration in Action   A first-grade class sorts fruit by color, texture, and size, giggling over "bumpy" oranges and "smooth" watermelon skin while practicing math and vocabulary. By fourth grade, they measure how much bread dough rises, blending science and math through play. In high school, that same approach grows into analyzing food marketing and media messages, real-world skills they'll actually use.

Why it works: Food lessons grow step by step, right alongside how kids think and learn. They meet kids where they are instead of jumping ahead with abstract or fear-based messages.

Body Positive in Schools

Students thrive when lessons shift the focus away from rules and shame and toward the idea that all bodies are good bodies and all foods have value. That might look like showing body diversity in books, celebrating cultural food traditions, or simply normalizing hunger and fullness cues. When this happens, kids feel: *My body is respected. I can trust myself.*

Food Exploration in Action   Second graders gather on the rug for a story about how bodies come in all shapes, sizes, and abilities. In middle school, students notice how different foods make them feel during a "tuning-in" project about energy, focus, and mood. By high school, cooking projects highlight food traditions from their own families and others, showing that all foods and all bodies belong.

> **Why it works:** Kids grow up trusting their bodies, celebrating differences, and questioning diet culture instead of carrying shame or comparison.

Experience-Based + Joyful in Schools

Kids learn best when food education feels more like a science lab or art studio than a worksheet. Planting seeds in the garden, tasting a new fruit in the cafeteria, or describing a carrot as "crunchy and sweet" instead of healthy turns food into meaningful, sensory-rich learning. When schools make space for hands-on exploration, kids think: *Food is fun. I want to explore more.*

Food Exploration in Action   Kindergarteners wrinkle their noses or smile as they smell mystery spices in jars and share what they remind them of. In art class, third graders use celery and Brussels sprouts to stamp colorful bouquets. Middle schoolers test their problem-solving skills with an assignment on "sketch or design a gadget that would make cooking easier for you." While high schoolers produce and edit short videos debunking food myths for health class.

> **Why it works:** Multi-sensory, hands-on lessons stick. They're fun, playful, and the ones kids remember long after the worksheets are forgotten.

Inclusive in Schools

Food education is strongest when it reflects the real diversity of the classroom. That means valuing tortillas, rice, and plantains as much as quinoa and kale, making safe foods available for kids with allergies or feeding challenges, and celebrating the food stories every child carries. When classrooms honor these differences, kids feel: My *story is valued. I belong here.*

Food Exploration in Action   In fourth grade, students create a "food globe," mapping family dishes from around the world. A second grader beams as she adds her grandmother's fried rice. In the cafeteria, taste-tests feature cultural dishes from different holidays throughout the calendar year alongside familiar favorites, always with the option to pass so everyone feels safe.

Why it works: When every child's food and body are honored, classrooms become places of pride, belonging, and genuine curiosity about others.

When food exploration drives learning, kids don't just remember the facts, they become moments to grow that last far beyond the classroom.

How Schools Can Make These Changes

Educational settings don't need to overhaul everything to make food and body lessons safer for kids—most don't have the resources to do so anyway. Even small, intentional shifts can make a meaningful difference: matching lessons to children's developmental stage, offering hands-on and practical experiences, and evaluating lessons for messages that may shame certain foods or bodies before teaching them.

> "Any classroom that employs a holistic model of learning will also be a place where teachers grow, and are empowered by the process."
>
> —bell hooks, *Teaching to Transgress*

Importantly, these shifts don't mean abandoning health education requirements. With thoughtful framing and support from passionate parents and health professionals, educators can still meet state standards—covering essential topics like nutrition, hydration, and balanced eating—while doing so in ways that reduce stigma, and spark curiosity rather than fear.

Food education can also be tailored to reflect the students a school serves. That might mean honoring cultural food traditions, acknowledging differences in food access, or supporting neurodivergent and sensory-sensitive learners. When children see their own experiences reflected in the classroom, lessons feel relevant and affirming, rather than distant or judgmental.

Reframing Food Education

Instead of. . .	Try this instead. . .
Sorting foods as "healthy" versus "unhealthy"	Sort foods by fruit types (e.g., pepo, drupe, berry) or veggie types (e.g., roots, stems, leaves) to build curiosity and pattern recognition. (*Experience-Based + Joyful*)
Using BMI report cards to talk about health	Talk about all the amazing things bodies can do. Teach Body Respect and care from a place of kindness, not shame. (*Body Positive*)
Calorie math or "burning off" food through exercise	Explore how different foods fuel different types of play (e.g., running, building, painting). Connect food to joyful movement. (*Experience-Based + Joyful*)
Praising kids for "clean plates" or trying bites for rewards	Let kids explore food with their senses, even if they don't eat it. Say: "You can just smell or touch it if you want." (*Experience-Based + Joyful*)
Asking kids to draw a "healthy plate" with limited foods	Invite kids to draw their family's favorite meal and share stories about it. Highlight connection and meaning. (*Inclusive*)

Partnering with Schools on Food and Nutrition Lessons

If you've been harmed by diet culture, it's natural to feel protective when your child starts receiving food and body lessons at school.

This concern is especially important in the elementary years, when your child's Food Positivity Protective Shield is still under construction, or for older children who haven't yet had the support they need to develop their Protective Shield.

The most important thing to remember is that teachers want the best for their students but usually have little control over the curriculum. Most health lessons come from district-approved materials, and many state standards specifically require teaching children to identify "healthy" versus "unhealthy" foods and "appropriate" portion sizes.

With that in mind, you can protect your child while also advocating for broader change. When you meet your child's teacher at the start of the school year or during a parent–teacher conference, let them know that developmentally appropriate food lessons and eating disorder prevention are priorities for your family. Teachers value knowing what matters to parents early on, especially when it's framed as protecting your child rather than critiquing their teaching.

You can make this easier for teachers by sharing our **Teacher One-Pager** with them. Let your teacher know that if they're expected to cover those topics, you'd appreciate a heads-up so you can decide whether to opt your child out.

These lessons also often show up in physical education (P.E.) classes as part of required health instruction, so consider sharing the **Teacher One-Pager** with your school's administration as well and asking about options to opt your child out of specific P.E.-based health lessons.

Bonus Handout via the QR Code: A Parent's One-Pager for Teachers

If you'd like to see broader change in how food and body lessons are taught at your school, the most effective place to raise concerns is with the district or school board. They're the ones deciding which curricula to purchase and pass along to teachers, which means that's where parent voices can directly influence what gets adopted for all students. Our **Advocating for District-Level Change** resource will help you navigate those bigger conversations.

Bonus Handout via the QR Code: Advocating for District-Level Change

Remember, the goal is never to tell teachers or administrators how to do their jobs. It's to protect your child, direct our advocacy to higher levels of the system where real change can happen, and keep the dialogue respectful while centering both educators' realities and children's well-being. By approaching educators with curiosity and collaboration, you create space for food and nutrition lessons that truly support every child.

Bringing It Home

You're not overreacting if your child's nutrition lessons feel off, confusing, or even potentially harmful. You're right to pause and ask questions. You now understand something that many nutrition education programs don't: that kids don't need more rules and charts to enjoy a variety of foods and build a healthy relationship with food and their bodies. They need safety, curiosity, and connection.

You've seen how nutrition education often misses the mark, not because people aren't trying but because the content and messaging haven't caught up with what we know about how kids learn. But now you have a new foundation to stand on. Food Positivity is a framework rooted in respect, science, and real life. We're not just teaching *about* food; we're using food to teach trust, identity, confidence, belonging and the life-ready skills they need to thrive.

And this is where change begins. When we bring these insights into conversations with schools, we open the door for education that reflects the Whole-Child, not just what's on their plate. We don't need to demand perfection, just a willingness to shift. Each small step away from shame and fear, toward curiosity and respect, helps create classrooms where children thrive—laying the groundwork for kids to carry trust in themselves and their bodies long after they leave the school setting.

One Simple Step

Today, notice just one nutrition message your child hears and reframe it together. When your child says something like "That food is bad," pause and invite a conversation.

Your Food Positivity Practice

Working with Your School for Positive Change

21

An Inclusive Whole-Child Approach to Healthcare

My son has always been big—big eyes, big heart, and a big body. Since birth, he has measured at or above the 99th percentile for height and weight, which has never bothered me. He rides his bike to school, spends hours playing outdoors and video games, and surprises people when he says his favorite food is mussels. For the past year and a half, we were called in to the pediatrician's office every three months for weigh-ins. In those visits, he overheard staff call him "obese." When he asked what that meant, the reply was, "It means you weigh too much." For weeks, he worried he was doing something wrong.

I carry my own history with body shame and disordered eating, and I don't want those same influences shaping him the way they shaped me. After each appointment I walk away defeated, racking my brain about whether my own experiences are clouding my judgment and wondering how this is affecting both of us.

—Bonnie

IF YOU'VE EVER left a medical setting feeling like your child's weight— whether high or low—overshadowed everything else, know that so many parents have felt that same knot in their stomach, wondering if their providers truly *saw* the child in front of them.

In Part I, we explored how body size itself does not determine much about someone's health and how poverty, racism, and the other

SDoH make it much harder for some many families to pursue true well-being, regardless of their body size.

But your child's medical professionals—and perhaps also you—may not yet be entirely convinced of this reality, and that's okay. We have all been trained to view weight as central to health. Over the last several decades, headlines about a "childhood obesity epidemic" have framed children's bodies as a crisis and pressured health professionals to act urgently.

Most medical training programs—and yes, this includes dietitians—just don't prepare providers to recognize weight stigma or practice from a place of Body Respect. When a child's weight falls above or below a line on the growth chart, many providers default to advice about food and exercise rooted in pressure and restriction—approaches that ignore genetics, food access, stress, and other powerful influences on health.

The result? You walk away feeling judged instead of supported. And mothers and caregivers in larger bodies often shoulder even *more* blame for their child's size or eating habits. So if you've ever felt that sting, it certainly doesn't mean you're failing as a parent—it means the system is failing *you* by ignoring the bigger picture of your child's well-being.

We know most providers genuinely care about kids, just like educators do. Once again, the real issue is the larger system that places weight—and a narrow, biased definition of "healthy" eating—at the center of pediatric care.

And we also don't want to dismiss the concerns *you* may have about your child's weight. Even if your child is thriving, it's normal to worry that they'll still face challenges because of society's perception of their body size or what they eat. What matters most, though, isn't their weight or percentile—it's whether they're growing along their own curve and supported in ways that honor their whole well-being, including the foods they love.

These worries are a reflection of just how much you care. And they put you in the perfect position to be your child's advocate, helping them feel safe, respected, and confident in their body. Let's explore the many issues that weight-focused healthcare creates and what truly supportive healthcare could look like for your child.

EXPERT INSIGHT: Pediatric Health Is More Than Meets the Eye

Jill Castle, MS, RDN of @ i.am.pedird, author of *Kids Thrive at Every Size* (Workman 2024), and The Nourished Child podcast

Healthcare providers may hone in on the appearance or size of a child and assume they are unhealthy. When this happens, we may unintentionally harm a child's emotional well-being, potentially negatively affecting their other areas of health and well-being. It's important to keep in mind that children are changing quite a bit, physically and emotionally, throughout the course of childhood. One of the best things we can do to protect their health and happiness is to focus on building the positive lifestyle habits that nurture a child's whole health. When food is nourishing, feeding is productive and positive, movement is fun, sleep is restorative, and families are deeply connected and supportive, children may grow up healthy and happy, at every size.

How Weight-Centric Care Misses the Mark

Healthcare that focuses on linking health to body size, uses BMI to predict disease risk, and prescribes weight loss is what's known as *weight-centric care*. And while it's hard enough to leave a medical visit feeling judged, what's worse is realizing that approaches built around changing a child's body size actually *fail* to help our kids thrive. They even create new risks, like the yo-yo dieting, eating disorders, and weight stigma we explored in Chapter 3.

And when these risks start in childhood, the harms can last a lifetime. Restrictive eating during a child's growing years can interfere with normal development, disrupt puberty, and lead to nutrient deficiencies. And because adolescence is already a peak risk period for eating disorders, making weight the issue only raises that likelihood.

You can support your child through strengthening their Food Positivity Protective Shield, but you can also advocate for quality healthcare for your child. Let's look at the specific harms of weight-centric care.

It Teaches Kids Their Bodies Are a Problem

When kids hear anyone talk about their weight negatively—whether too high or too low—they learn to see their body as the problem. But when those words come from a medical professional, the message hits even harder. And even when professionals offer these insights with the health of the child in mind, research shows that *any* weight talk or dieting advice in front of the child raises the risk of eating disorders and future weight gain.

As a result, children may begin to feel ashamed of their bodies, avoid foods they once enjoyed, or even start to question whether you see them the same way.

> As the provider looks over a child's chart, they say, "You're awfully small for your age." The words echo in the child's mind, and later at school they compare themselves to their classmates, suddenly noticing how much taller and stronger everyone else seems.

It Ignores Child Development and Autonomy

Even children above the ninety-fifth percentile may be completely healthy if their growth is steady, labs are normal, and development is on track. But when providers tell them they're eating "too much," "not enough," or need to "watch their weight," it assumes they have the skills to monitor food the way adults do (though in truth, that kind of monitoring isn't realistic or healthy for most adults either). Kids don't have the ability to take on that responsibility—and they shouldn't have to anyway.

When health advice skips over their developmental needs, kids lose trust in both their caregivers and their own bodies.

> A provider asks a child about their favorite foods. They eagerly list ice cream and spaghetti, and the provider says, "Just be careful not to eat too many carbs." Later, the child starts asking which foods have carbs and avoiding some of their most loved dishes.

It Sends the Message That Families Are at Fault

Too often, weight-focused care leaves parents feeling like they've failed their child. Providers may criticize a child's eating habits without considering factors like access, stress, culture, or genetics. And these comments generally aren't paired with meaningful support or guidance.

A family's everyday meals may be nourishing, familiar, and highly meaningful, but if they don't match their provider's narrow picture of health (hello, healthism), families leave feeling judged instead of supported.

When a provider's advice doesn't include meaningful support and guidance, families leave feeling judged rather than supported.

> At a check-up, the provider asks what foods the mother usually buys. When she mentions frozen pizza and cereal, the provider sighs and says, "Well, that explains it." She leaves feeling judged and blamed, even though those choices fit her budget and schedule.

It Centers Compliance, Not Care or Curiosity

Weight-focused care tends to turn health to rules: "Eat this, not that," or "Exercise more." This pressure often comes from the biased assumption that families need stricter rules, when what they really need is partnership and guidance that respects their child's needs.

Over time, parents and kids may begin to dread and avoid visits, and that fear can keep them from getting help when they truly need it.

> At a toddler's follow-up, the provider notes they haven't gained any weight since the last visit, despite the family being instructed to serve calorie-dense meals. The parent had tried to follow that advice and endured mealtime battles as a result but leaves feeling like they've failed.

It Misses the Opportunity for Truly Supportive Care

When providers focus on weight, families lose the chance to talk about what would really help their child. Important steps like screening for food insecurity, stress, or sleep issues or offering referrals and support for routines around meals and movement often get skipped in favor of focusing on the child's body.

As a result, families walk away without the care and resources that could make a real difference.

> A parent mentions they're concerned about their child's sudden weight gain and constant fatigue. The provider tells them to "watch portions" and "get more exercise" without running labs that would indicate the need for a referral to endocrinology for a hypothyroidism diagnosis.

Provider Bias: A Real Issue in Pediatric Care

Most providers go into every visit with the goal of helping kids grow and thrive. But even the most caring professionals can still practice under the influence of harmful biases—a reality research continues to highlight.

Studies show that many providers believe people can control their weights and that they think recommending weight loss is safe, despite a lot of evidence to the contrary. Research also shows that providers often spend less time with patients in larger bodies, offer fewer treatment options, and sometimes even show less respect.

Bias isn't always intentional, but it has real consequences, and you and your family have the right to inclusive, patient-centered care.

Weight-Inclusive Care: A Different Approach to Health

We hope you feel confident by now that we're not denying the very real health challenges kids face today. But those challenges are so much bigger than diet and body size alone—they're rooted in inequity and a deep need for caregivers who can guide and support children to thrive. In medical settings, that kind of support has a name: *weight-inclusive care.*

When you're working with a weight-inclusive provider, you can be confident that they won't judge your child's health by their size. They'll look at the whole child: growth patterns, food access, labs, sleep, mental health, and home life. They'll use respectful, neutral language and focus on habits that truly support well-being: shared meals, balanced routines, joyful movement, and positive body image. They'll still track a child's weight trends, but it will be just one data point in the bigger picture of your child's health, not the entire story.

Depending on where you live or what your insurance covers, weight-inclusive care may be hard to find. It might take extra questions, referrals, or even trial and error to find someone who truly centers your child's well-being over their weight—tasks you likely don't have time for! But even knowing what this kind of care looks like can help you recognize it when you see it and advocate for it when you don't.

Here's a side-by-side look at how weight-centric and weight-inclusive care handle common parts of a child's medical visit—and what each approach communicates to children and families.

Element of Pediatric Care	Weight-Centric Approach	Weight-Inclusive Approach
Medical Language	Terms like "obese" or "underweight" come from training and guidelines but often feel stigmatizing.	Providers use neutral, respectful language (e.g., high or low body weight) to protect dignity and Body Trust.
Growth Monitoring	Growth charts and BMI percentiles are often treated as a primary indicator of health. Families of children above or below certain ranges may be advised with strategies to change their body size.	Growth charts are used to look at patterns over time and check for changes that may indicate underlying issues. Weight is treated as one piece of health, alongside labs, development, and family context.

(continued)

(*continued*)

Element of Pediatric Care	Weight-Centric Approach	Weight-Inclusive Approach
Response to Eating Concerns	Weight loss in larger kids may be praised, even if caused by restriction. Struggles in smaller kids may be dismissed as "just picky."	Providers create space for open, stigma-free conversations about eating behaviors and screen for disordered eating regardless of body size.
Overall Goal of Care	Success is often framed as moving toward the "middle" of the chart, with weight change as the main outcome.	Success means helping kids grow into their natural, genetic size while building a healthy relationship with food and their bodies.

A Better Way Forward

When we think about what truly supports kids' health, it's clear that shrinking their bodies isn't the answer. What *does* make a difference is care that meets kids where they are. Weight-inclusive care has been shown to improve measurable health markers like blood pressure and cholesterol, while also boosting mental health and body image. The best part? These benefits show up regardless of what happens with a child's weight.

> "*I believe that the basis of any health education lies in a person's caring enough about himself that he'll want to take care of himself. If we want people to eat the right food, brush their teeth, get the proper exercise, seek regular checkups. . .we must help these people feel that they're really worth taking care of.*"
>
> —Fred Rogers, *You Are Special*

And compared to weight-centric care—which often *increases* the risks it aims to prevent—weight-inclusive care does the opposite. It reduces the chance of disordered eating, helps kids build a trusting relationship with food, and encourages lifelong self-care—everything we're after with Food Positivity. And just like education, the whole-child is at the heart of Food Positive medical care. Every appointment becomes a chance for you to feel heard, respected, and backed up as your child's best advocate.

The Food Positivity Learning Foundations in Healthcare

The good news is that many providers are already moving in a direction that aligns with the Food Positivity Learning Foundations. In fact, over the last several decades, the Health at Every Size™ (HAES) model has helped support exactly this type of shift by offering a framework that centers well-being over weight and helps providers better support children—and adults—of all sizes. It encourages medical care that is respectful and stigma-free and supports the child's overall health, whatever size their body happens to be.

To show you how this approach aligns with Food Positivity, we've adapted the best practices of weight-inclusive care to fit our Food Positivity Learning Foundations. Because just like with education, your child thrives when their medical care reflects the following principles.

Developmentally Attuned in Healthcare

Kids' needs change as their bodies, brains, and emotions grow and a parent's role shifts right along with them. At some stages, kids need parents to take the lead, providing structure and reassurance. At others, they need space to speak for themselves, with parents offering support in the background. When healthcare reflects both the child's stage and the parent's evolving role, families feel: *This plan makes sense for us.*

Body Positive in Healthcare

Families thrive when providers affirm their worth at every appointment. Care that avoids judgment and celebrates body diversity helps children see their bodies as capable and deserving of respect. When providers focus on strengths, use neutral language, and encourage confidence over shame, families hear: *Care is collaborative. Our voice matters.*

Experience-Based + Joyful in Healthcare

Families don't just need instructions; they need care that meets them where they are. That means listening to their stories, honoring what already works, and suggesting small, realistic changes that feel doable. When providers share guidance through curiosity and partnership, celebrate progress, and connect families to the right support, the message is clear: *Our healthcare experience is important. We can work on our health as a team.*

Inclusive in Healthcare

Every family carries their own story, shaped by culture, resources, and lived realities. Healthcare that respects those differences by acknowledging systemic barriers, honoring traditions, and recognizing natural body diversity helps families feel safe and valued. In those moments, families hear: *Our culture is valued. We belong here just as we are.*

EXPERT INSIGHT: Cultural Humility in Healthcare

Tamara S. Melton, MS, RDN, LD of @tamarameltonrdn and Co-Founder and Executive Director of Diversify Dietetics

Advocating for Culturally Humble Care

Your child's healthcare providers have expertise in their fields of practice, but you bring expertise too. You know your family's culture, values, and daily life. *Cultural humility* means that a provider recognizes this and approaches care with curiosity and respect, not assumptions. It's the ongoing practice of listening, learning, and adjusting care to honor each family's lived experience.

A culturally humble provider might ask questions like, "What foods are important in your family?" or "Where do you usually shop or eat?" instead of simply saying what your child *should* eat.

They use your insights to shape care that actually fits your family. That's your right as a parent—and if a provider doesn't yet have that awareness, it's their responsibility to learn it.

If a comment about your child's body or eating habits feels off, ask, *"What did you mean by that?"* or *"How does that relate to my child's health?"* They should be able to explain their reasoning clearly, just like they would for an ear infection or vaccination.

Remember, kids notice everything: tone, body language, even what's left unsaid. When you speak up or check in after an uncomfortable moment, you're not just advocating for your child's care; you're showing them how to advocate for themselves. Cultural humility isn't just for healthcare—it's a life skill. By modeling it, you help your child grow into an adult who expects and gives respect in every space they enter.

Partnering with Providers on Your Child's Care

Your instincts matter when it comes to your child's medical care. Pediatric visits should feel safe, respectful, and focused on your child's needs, not shaming or overwhelming. This kind of care has a name: empathetic, trauma-informed, patient-centered care.

One of the best ways to set this tone is by being clear about your expectations early. You can let your provider know that you'd like any discussion of weight or food choices to happen without your child present, especially when they're young and still building their Food Positivity Protective Shield. Keeping kids out of sensitive conversations in medical settings isn't overprotective—it's developmentally appropriate. You can also ask for "blind weights," where the provider records your child's weight but does not share the number with them.

You can expect your provider to see the full picture of your child's health. And if their focus feels too specific to your child's size or eating habits, you have every right to gently redirect the conversation.

If your provider's care doesn't feel balanced or respectful, you still have options. You might ask more questions, request a second opinion, or clarify what kind of support you need. And if their care still doesn't feel supportive, it's okay to seek a provider who's a better fit for your family's needs and values. Of course, not every family has the privilege of switching providers. If that's your situation, remember that *you* still have the final say in your child's medical care—and that the supportive home environment you're building is what matters most in shaping your child's relationship with food and their body.

Bringing It Home

No parent should have to walk into a medical visit bracing for judgment. And no child should walk out believing their body is a problem. You and your child deserve care that affirms their worth, respects *your* role as a parent, and offers meaningful guidance that truly supports health.

You are your child's best advocate. By seeking out weight-inclusive, patient-centered care and setting clear boundaries with your providers, you not only protect your child's well-being today but also show them the kind of medical care they deserve for years to come.

As with our parenting and education approaches, change in medical settings begins when we stop centering weight and rigid ideas about "healthy" behaviors and start centering children and their individual challenges and needs. We can push the system to do better. Providers who choose curiosity over judgment create safer spaces for kids to grow into Food Positivity. Together, families and providers can move medical care toward a future where it nurtures confidence, health, and dignity for every child.

One Simple Step

Before your child's next appointment, write down a short list of the things you want to focus on with your provider, like your child's sleep, stress, or your specific concerns about their health. Start the visit by asking them to partner with you on your child's overall well-being and the list you've brought.

Your Food Positivity Practice
Medical Conversations Made Easier: *Small Shifts to Build Confidence*

22

Raising the Next Generation to Be SAFE

Your child is now a teen. Out with her friends, she orders a burger and fries. Someone who ordered a salad says, "Are you really going to eat all that?" She jokes back, "Hey, eyes on your own plate!" and enjoys her meal. She doesn't quite finish it though, because she and another friend had talked about splitting a chocolate lava cake and she wants to save room.

She's starting to like salad at home, but reminds you to buy the kits without cabbage because her favorite is Caesar. She often fixes her own snacks—her latest creation was baba ghanoush—but tends to arrive hungry for the dinners you make and regularly suggests new recipes you can cook together.

You're in awe of her confidence. Her clothes and personal style embody her individuality in ways you never would have dreamed of as a teen yourself. Sometimes she has self-doubts—often because of what her friends are doing or things she sees online—but she knows she can always come to you to chat over a pint of ice cream. This is Food Positivity.

You've come a long way.

If you've made it to this chapter, it means you've sat with hard truths about diet culture, reflected on your own food and body story, and practiced new ways of talking and showing up at the table. That's no small thing. It takes courage to face the grief of what you didn't receive as a child, the guilt that bubbles up when you slip into old patterns, and the hope of doing things differently for your kids, however imperfectly.

Let's be honest, it's hard work to parent against the grain of a culture that constantly tells us what body sizes are best, that our body cues are untrustworthy, and that good parenting requires control and obedience. If it has felt lonely or exhausting at times, we are right there with you. You are doing something radical and deeply protective.

Know that you've already done such meaningful work by reading this book. We know that you may not feel like you fully grasp how to put all of these strategies into practice yet—and that's more than okay. No parent comes away from one book with it all figured out—or more accurately, no parent has it all figured out, ever. Our workbook *Food Positivity Practice: A Guided Playbook for Real-Life Parenting* will help you translate this new way forward into your daily life, with joy, confidence, and connection. What matters most is that you're showing up, reflecting, and willing to see things differently. Even when it hasn't felt like you're doing everything "right," you've been shifting the ground your kids stand on, and that matters.

Unlearning and Healing Is Yours to Claim

Supporting your child in developing Food Positivity also means taking a look inward. The Modeling, Messaging, and everyday Moments that shape their relationship with food and their bodies are influenced by the relationship *you* have with food and your body, the Family Core Values that guide your decisions, and even the way you process your own emotions. Every bit of work you do here benefits both you and your child—in body, mind, and spirit.

You may not feel ready to take on that kind of personal work, and that's completely understandable. Facing your own food story can feel overwhelming, especially in a culture that still treats body size as a marker of worth and health. Maybe you're hoping your child will learn to eat intuitively and embrace their body, even while you quietly lean on familiar patterns of control or conformity for yourself, simply because that feels safer right now. Or maybe you truly want to become an adult who nourishes yourself with ease, regardless of your body size, but you're still just not sure how to step away from years of diet culture. You get to pick what feels best to you. Wherever you are, know this: even small, imperfect steps toward Food Positivity will strengthen your own inner voice and ripple outward to benefit your family.

> "We have the power to change the narrative of body shame in our lives. We are not bound to the tales of teasing and criticism we were subjected to as children. The good news is we are the authors of our own lives."
> —Sonya Renee Taylor, *The Body Is Not an Apology*

You might consider working with a nutrition professional trained in eating disorder recovery, Intuitive Eating, or responsive feeding. And honestly, what parent wouldn't benefit from a good therapist these days? A mental health provider can help you sort through the values you were raised with—or simply absorbed from a culture that glorifies self-sacrifice and body ideals. Doing this work can bring you more peace with food and give you the freedom to model something different for your child.

We know the push for positivity can feel toxic at times, and that's not at all what we're encouraging. You don't have to love your body or feel great about your food choices all the time. Perfect is the enemy of the good, and the last thing we want is for you to turn these ideas into another set of rigid rules. As you've seen, none of this is about trading diet culture's rules for new ones. It's about building a foundation rooted in safety, trust, connection, and true well-being.

Your child doesn't need you to "get it right" all the time. What they need most is a parent who is willing to keep learning, reflecting, and healing right alongside them.

From the Big Picture to Everyday Moments

This book has taken you on a journey. We started by peeling back the curtain on diet culture—how it shaped the food system, our definitions of health, and the way so many of us talk to kids. We explored how children actually learn about food and bodies—not through lectures or rules—but through experiences, relationships, and age-appropriate development and support. We looked at how your own food story intersects with theirs, and we practiced scripts and strategies for those tricky everyday moments: dessert demands, body comments, family pressure, and more.

In the past few chapters, we zoomed out to the bigger picture of schools, healthcare, and culture, because raising kids free from food and body shame happens in a dynamic world—one we hope to partner with you on in changing for the better. And now, we'll zoom back in. Back to you, your kids, and your table.

Supporting your child well starts with truly knowing them well. Helping them nourish their body is important, no doubt, but our work as parents has always been much bigger than "just nutrition." Food Positivity is about raising kids who trust their bodies, who are comfortable with a variety of foods, and who leave our homes one day confident in the Life Skills that will carry them forward—skills of self-trust, flexibility, joy, and connection that shape not just how they eat but how they live. And that starts with understanding your child's whole world—their brain, body, beliefs, and needs—so you can respond to the whole person they already are.

At its heart, feeding isn't just about food. It's about your relationship with your child, shaped by all the experiences you've had with food and your body yourself. And while this role is rewarding, it's also deeply challenging, because it asks you to bring your best self to a process that unfolds multiple times every single day.

SAFE is a tool to help take that weight off your shoulders. It's a simple, memorable tool you can lean on when you feel stuck, reminding you of the foundations you've already been building.

From Framework to Compass: SAFE A Simple Approach for Positive Food and Body Learning

The Food Positivity Framework you've worked through in these chapters is the map, a way to understand the bumpy terrain of raising kids in a diet culture world. Your Family Core Values are the compass, the north star, that points you in the direction you want for your family long-term.

But in the middle of an actual mealtime meltdown or a tough question at the doctor's office, pulling out a whole map can feel overwhelming. SAFE is your pocket compass, the simple, memorable approach for positive food and body learning you can grab when you feel stuck. It distills everything we've covered into four guiding points that remind you what matters most and show you the next step:

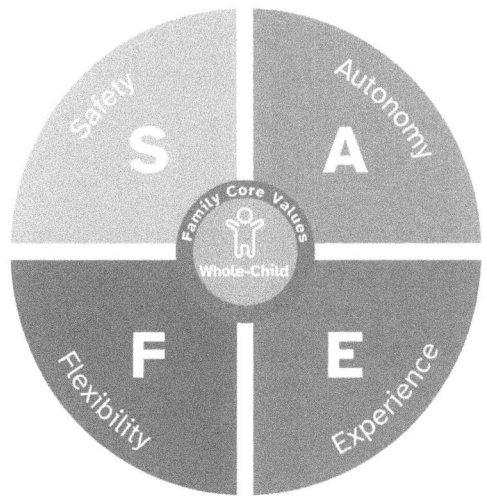

S = Safety—Kids can only learn when they feel physically, emotionally, and socially safe.

A = Autonomy—Children need voice and choice to build trust in their bodies and cues.

F = Flexibility—Growth isn't linear; regressions are normal. Meet kids where they are.

E = Experience—Real learning comes through doing: tasting, touching, stirring, squishing, smelling, and living.

SAFE isn't a checklist, it's a gut-check. It creates a protective, responsive foundation for food and body learning. When things feel messy, you can ask yourself: *Am I offering Safety, Autonomy, Flexibility, or Experience here?* Even one letter is enough to shift the moment.

What SAFE Looks Like

Safety means your child feels calm and cared for, not pressured or judged.

> **Scenario:** At a birthday party, instead of hovering as your child takes a cupcake, you might simply say, "I'm here if you need me." That steady presence keeps their nervous system regulated.
>
> **Script:** "Enjoy the cupcake! If your body says you've had enough for now, I can keep it safe for you so you can enjoy the rest later!"
>
> **Food Positivity Framework:** In one small moment, you're practicing every Guiding Need—staying Attuned by noticing what your child is really asking for, bringing a Calm + Steady Presence to keep the moment low-pressure, and showing Body Respect by honoring their signals.

Autonomy means your child has a say in what happens to their body.

> **Scenario:** Your child refuses broccoli but asks for another scoop of potatoes. Instead of insisting, you smile and say, "Help yourself," and hand them the spoon. In that moment, you're guiding food learning in a way that helps them feel respected and valued at the table.
>
> **Script:** "Your body, your choice. You decide what goes on your fork."
>
> **Food Positivity Framework:** In one small moment, you're practicing every Guiding Skill—being Developmentally Attuned by offering choice that fits their stage, teaching through a Body Positive lens by honoring their cues, creating an Inclusive environment by validating their preferences, and making food Experience-Based + Joyful by inviting them to serve themselves.

Flexibility means remembering that kids don't grow in straight lines.

> **Scenario:** Maybe your adventurous eater suddenly only wants buttered noodles. You remind yourself, "When parents offer consistent meals with a variety of foods, kids typically get what they need to grow and thrive." By offering noodles with a side of fruit

and veggies and enjoying them yourself, you keep variety present without pressure.

Script: "What was the best part of your day? Let's share a 'rose and thorn' (best and hardest part of the day)."

Food Positivity Framework: In one small moment, you're aligning your Invisible Curriculum 3 Ms: Modeling by enjoying the same meal, shifting the Message away from food talk, and creating a safe Moment of connection where food feels flexible instead of forced. And that's what helps kids relax and stay open to food at their own pace.

Experience means kids learn through doing, not being told.

Scenario: At the store, your child spots a carambola (starfruit) that they've never seen before. You show them how to pick out the best one, lifting the fruit to their nose so they can smell the light floral aroma and add it to the cart, telling them, "When we get home, we're going to be Food Explorers!" Later, you cut it open together and notice how each slice is in the shape of a star, how the skin is yellow and waxy, and when you slice it open, how the juicy flesh has a similar texture to a grape.

Script: "We are Food Explorers in search of delicious! Let's use our five senses to learn more about this fruit. What do you notice?"

Food Positivity Framework: In one small moment, you're bridging all the Growing Skills of the Learning Foundations into practicing by sparking your child's natural curiosity with Food Exploration. By making space for child-led, hands-on discovery, you're helping your child build confidence and trust through real experiences instead of rules.

SAFE in Everyday Life

SAFE isn't just for your kitchen table; it's for the world your child is growing up in.

- **At the doctor's office:** *Safety* might mean stepping in if a provider comments on your child's weight while they are present.

"We're focusing on eating foods that help our bodies feel best and feel joyful, not numbers." That protects their Felt Safety.

- **At a family gathering:** *Autonomy* might mean letting your child politely decline Aunt Linda's spinach pie without jumping in to smooth it over because their voice, their no, matters.
- **At school:** *Flexibility* might mean sending your kiddo with a chocolate milk and their favorite packed snacks because that's what helps them fill their belly in the busy lunchroom with big smells and plan for a bigger afternoon mini-meal snack when they get home because you are Attuning to their needs.
- **At a playdate:** *Experience* might mean inviting kids to make their own snack mix from bowls on the counter with pretzels, raisins, seeds, and chocolate chips, turning an ordinary snack time into a fun snacktivity.

SAFE travels with you wherever you go. It's not about doing everything right. It's about having a simple compass in your pocket that points you toward connection, trust, and growth.

A Whole-SAFE Moment

You're at a family dinner; the full table is loud, and you can start to feel your mealtime tension building. Your child refuses the main dish and starts reaching for only bread rolls. You feel the old panic rising: *They need more than carbs!* You pause and check your pocket compass.

- **Safety:** You take a breath, soften your tone, and say, "Looks like you found something you like."
- **Autonomy:** You say nothing when they grab two rolls and a giant scoop of butter on their plate as they walk toward you.
- **Flexibility:** You remind yourself that this one meal won't make or break meeting their nutrient needs, and tomorrow you can offer more variety in a space that feels safe.
- **Experience:** You show them how to slice open the roll and spread the butter and invite them to do the same for the other roll. You may even suggest that they offer to butter the rolls for other family members, keeping them engaged with the family and the food in a low-pressure way.

Instead of the moment spiraling into a battle, you've stayed SAFE. That's the power of this compass.

SAFE Is Enough

By now, you've noticed: SAFE doesn't ask you for perfection; it asks you for presence. Even the tiniest SAFE shifts plant seeds of trust your child carries forward. SAFE is enough. And so are you.

You're Healing Too

As you practice SAFE, you may notice that you're offering your kids what you didn't get. That can feel bittersweet, both healing and heavy. Remember, this is your journey too. Every SAFE choice you make isn't just raising a child who trusts their body, it's repairing the part of you that needed the same care and that healing matters.

The Power of Community

This work is lighter when it's shared. Start where you are: invite a friend to read this book with you and talk about the "aha" moments. Form a parent group or book club where Food Positivity becomes shared language. Connect with online communities that celebrate body diversity and anti-diet parenting. Bring SAFE and Food Positivity into your child's school or pediatrician's office. Food Positivity isn't just for your home, it's a cultural shift we build together. When parents choose it collectively, schools become safer, doctors more compassionate, and communities more inclusive.

Bringing It Home

Your kids don't need perfect meals, perfect words, or perfect parents. What they need is you, present, caring, and willing to grow alongside them. And you are already giving your child a different story.

Food Positivity is more than a framework. It's a way of raising children who trust their bodies, who know they belong, and who can move through the world free from food and body shame. SAFE may be your pocket compass, but your Family Core Values remain your true north, guiding your everyday choices and your family's long-term vision.

Your lasting legacy is in the everyday small shifts you make because it doesn't just protect your child today but strengthens their Protective Shield and the foundation for the next generation. Every time you pause instead of pressuring, reflect instead of reacting, or choose connection over control, you're supporting your child to develop the kind of relationship with food and bodies we all truly deserve.

Your children will carry this trust into their own families, their communities, and, yes, even into how they raise their children one day.

Together, we are raising the first generation free from food and body shame and starting a ripple that will reshape the future our kids inherit. And it starts here, with you.

One Simple Step
When in doubt, come back to SAFE. Even one letter is enough.

Your Food Positivity Practice
SAFE: *Your Pocket Compass for Food Positivity*

Acknowledgments

Diana:

I would like to thank every client who has ever shared their heart with me and every member of Raising Anti-Diet Kids. Your questions and insights have inspired every page of this book. Thank you for doing the hard work to break the cycle of food and body shame and craft a better future for our children. Because of your commitment, your children will not suffer as you have, and that is the greatest gift you can give them. I am especially grateful to the many professional colleagues from whom I have learned this approach and the many body liberation educators and activists who have humbled me with their insights and dedication to creating a world where everyBODY is valued. Thank you to my colleagues at The Collective who have supported me through all the ups and downs, and of course, thank you to my incredible husband and amazingly creative and insightful daughters, without whom this book would not have been possible.

Dani:

To my husband, Michael, you are one of a kind. Thank you for your unwavering love, patience, and belief in me. This book wouldn't have been possible without you.

To my girls, you are the meaning of joy. Thank you for your love and patience while Mama worked to help kids around the world, even when it meant less time together. You'll always be my why.

To my best friend and illustrator, Mary, you are a gift. Thank you for being my creative partner, cheerleader, and steady source of light. I don't know what I'd do without you.

To the parents and educators who keep asking brave questions about how to raise kids differently, you are the reason this book exists.

And last, but never least, to the next generation: thank you for teaching us as we learn to heal ourselves. You are our future.

Index